FOREWORD

A s a woman in my early forties and a Clinical Nurse with over 23 years' experience, I have witnessed first-hand the transformative journey that women undergo as they navigate the often misunderstood and overlooked phase of menopause. It is with great empathy and understanding that I introduce this book by Mahesh Prabhu, which serves as a beacon of knowledge and support for women embarking on this significant chapter of their lives.

In a world of healthcare, pharmacists are the trusted guides who help us navigate the complexities of medication and wellness. I have known Mahesh for over 20 years and in that time, he has brought a wealth of knowledge and dedication to patient care. With his deep understanding of medication, supplements and a holistic approach to health, Mahesh brings a perspective that is both grounded in science and informed by compassion.

Menopause is not merely a biological event; it is a profound transition that encompasses physical, emotional, and psychological changes. Yet, despite its universality, menopause remains shrouded in stigma and misinformation. As a nurse, I have encountered countless women who grapple with uncertainty, discomfort, and even fear as they confront this natural progression.

Mahesh has written a comprehensive guide that seeks to demystify menopause and empower women to embrace this transition with grace and resilience. From understanding the hormonal shifts, to reducing the frequency and intensity of symptoms with a simple 4 – 6-week practical plan, this uncomplicated book gives woman the desire to complete the self-guided section in order to manage and overcome symptoms.

But beyond the clinical aspect, this book recognises the deeply personal and unique journey that each woman experiences during menopause. Through candid accounts and shared experiences, it honours the diversity of woman's narratives, acknowledging that no two journeys are alike.

As I reflect on my own journey through womanhood, I am reminded of the importance of knowledge, support, and solidarity. It is my hope that this book will serve as a trusted companion for women navigating the complexities of menopause, offering guidance, reassurance, and above all, the affirmation that they are not alone.

This book will be a source of empowerment, enlightenment, and encouragement for all women embarking on this transformative journey.

A. Rogan RN Western Australia

In the ever shifting and dynamic realm of healthcare, every professional is afforded the freedom to carve their own path. Mahesh Prabhu, a UK-based Pharmacist, has emerged as a beacon of hope and support for menopausal women globally. Our paths converged in a bustling Australian pharmacy in Queensland, where Mahesh was working after having recently migrated from the UK. His holistic approach to patient well-being has profoundly influenced my career trajectory, guiding my transition from an Enrolled Nurse to an aspiring Registered Nurse.

As I enter my early thirties as a woman, I have witnessed first-hand the significant impact of menopause—a phase often overlooked in discussions of womanhood. Observing the challenges faced by many women navigating this transition alone has strengthened my resolve to ensure better support for both myself and others in the future. My experiences as a nurse in Queensland, Australia, serve as the basis for this resolve.

This book offers invaluable insights that transcend conventional medical advice, providing illumination on the complexities of menopause with empathy and understanding. It recognises the uniqueness of each woman's journey and strives to be a steadfast companion during times of uncertainty. What particularly captivated me was its pragmatic, evidence-based approach to managing symptoms, with or without the use of medications. In an area where the default often leans towards a pill-based solution, finding evidence-based research for alternative treatments is uncommon. Engaging with this work not only promises enlightening "aha" moments but also offers the reassurance of companionship on this transformative journey.

A. Nolan RN Queensland, Australia

Dedication

To my wife Susan

meno pause *zen*

Mahesh V Prabhu BSc

INTRODUCTION

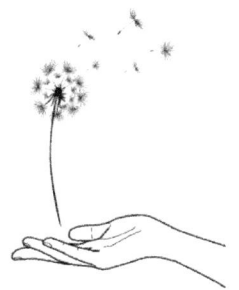

Menopause is a life-changing event that allows women to step into a new chapter of freedom, manage the ups and downs of change, and rediscover their strength within. This self-help book is more than just a list of words; it's designed to be a roadmap made to help you negotiate some of the more distressing aspects of menopause. In the next pages, you will find the compass to navigate the realms of hot flushes, night sweats, brain fog, fatigue, genitourinary symptoms, and joint pain with or without the use of medications including hormonal replacement therapy (HRT). Regaining the ability to shape the experiences rather than erasing them is the goal of this journey.

This book sets out a self-help programme where an individual symptom is tackled over a 4-6 week period. It is a guide encompassing elements of Cognitive Behavioural Therapy, Holistic Practices and Behavioural Changes which the reader can easily embrace and integrate into their daily lives. The book is ideal for women who refuse, or who are unable to take medications, as well as for those who are looking for alternative practices to lower their dosage including HRT. It is also a useful tool for those women experiencing menopausal style symptoms post-breast cancer.

The information provided within is split into two sections; **Knowledge**, where the reader gains a scientific insight behind the cause of some of their symptoms, and **Action,** where the reader uses multiple evidence-based practices to help obtain relief for a particular symptom over a 4-6 week period. Symptoms are monitored over the time period and practices are adjusted according to the relief obtained. An invaluable section is also included for men to help guide them and support the menopausal turbulence their partners or work colleagues may experience.

The online version of the book has been created into a self help, do at home digital programme which also includes video and audio elements that cannot be included in a book format such as hypnosis. The programme can be found at **www.sisstas.com**

Mahesh V Prabhu is a UK Pharmacist and certified by The British Menopause Society. He has over 25 years experience in both the UK and Australian healthcare systems. As a certified hypnotherapist and former obesity health practitioner with the World Obesity Federation, he has helped many men and women manage their health over the years including their weight and other chronic medical conditions.

CONTENTS

ILLUSTRATIONS

KNOWLEDGE

Welcome

"I see menopause as the start of the next fabulous phase of life as a woman. Now is a time to 'tune in' to our bodies and embrace this new chapter. If anything, I feel more myself and love my body more now, at 58 years old, than ever before."

– Actress Kim Cattrall

Menopause isn't just an ending; it's a beginning. It's a chance to understand what is happening to your body and embrace your inner strength and resilience. I would love for you to understand that the power is already in your hands, so please recognise it and give it back to yourself so you can accept an inevitable change, and make new plans for the future.

Hi, my name is Mahesh Prabhu and I have been a practising pharmacist since I first registered over 25 years ago in the United Kingdom. I have worked in both the United Kingdom and Australian healthcare systems and have found men and women the world over have the same health challenges facing them.

Even though we have made great advancements in technology and health-care, we are the most diseased we have ever been despite the billions ploughed in every year through government expenditure in every western country around the planet. How is this possible and why is there such a mismatch?

Over the years I have become more anti-medication as I see a never-ending list of medications being prescribed at every age group, and profit being made at every opportunity. It seems that whatever complaint we have around our health, there appears to be a tablet waiting to 'fix' it. Could it be that the best way to health and longevity is to manage our health without medications, as best as we can by going back to basics of good nutrition and movement, reviewing our work-life balance, and seeking alternative health practices?

Since the drug and prescription mantra seems to be so ingrained in our western culture, I wrote this book as an aid to help women looking for an alternative to hormone replacement therapy (HRT), or simply for those who cannot, or will not take HRT medication. There is much wisdom in alternative holistic practices. I am not here to denigrate HRT or push an antagonistic Big Pharma agenda. There will always be women who may fall under the high risk category or just those seeking an alternative path. This is for you.

When I was thinking about this self-help guide, I was determined not to come across as 'Mansplaining'. In other words, I wanted to avoid sounding condescending or patronising, especially considering that this is a very sensitive topic that primarily concerns women, even though it will cross a man's path in this area of female health. My intention is not to diminish or undermine anyone's expertise or experience in this area of health, but rather to provide opinion, knowledge, and insights through my own experience in the subject matter. From the numerous talks I have had with women over the years, I hope to be suggestive rather than prescriptive in my attempts to share the information here.

As mentioned previously, the book is split into two main sections, Knowledge and Action. The knowledge section is just a brief overview via short chapters of some of the main symptoms a woman may experience, and a little bit of science behind them. It would be impossible to cover all of the 40+ symptoms currently reported in this area, so I have decided to concentrate on the main ones that most women find distressing. The book's main idea is to focus on self-help rather than coming across as a biology lecture. There have been many other books written on menopause so you may already be wise to the information, or have read around the subject matter. If this is the case then please move on to the action section of the book. If not, then I wanted to keep things brief and as simple as I could without waffling on; I think there is plenty of advice and information out there already.

Whilst I didn't want to write a scientific paper, I think it is important to have a basic understanding of the background behind the symptoms. That being said, feel free to skip over the scientific explanations if you'd like; they serve merely to give a streamlined explanation of how and why the symptoms manifest.

I didn't want to write a publication with just advice and information. This book is more action-focused. The Action section gives you a framework on how to start tackling the main distressing areas which include hot flushes and night sweats, fatigue, brain fog, joint pain, and genito-urinary challenges.

There is an online version of this book which I have developed into a digital programme that includes elements that cannot be included in a book such as video and audio for example hypnosis. You can find this at **www.sisstas.com**

Each symptom is designed to be tackled alone over a 4-6 week period by taking massive determined action. This is about managing your symptoms so that your quality of life is significantly improved, and not necessarily a cure for them all. Medications can be added or removed at any point in this guide depending on your success rate.

You may be thinking, why would a male Pharmacist in his late 50s be helping a woman with menopausal symptoms?

What would he know about it!

Having practised here in the UK and abroad, I am quite surprised over the years just how many women have opened up to me when I provided a listening ear to them. I have had the privilege of interacting with numerous women who have shared their experiences and concerns about menopause, especially in light of how difficult it was to see their GP. This has allowed me to gain a deeper understanding of the challenges they face and the importance of someone just being there for them when they needed professional support.

I guess most people just see me as another health professional and usually just like to pick my brain a little and vent.

My background equips me with a deep understanding of medications, therapies, and health-related issues. This has allowed me to provide valuable, evidence-based advice to women experiencing menopausal symptoms as well as help women make informed decisions about treatment options, both pharmacological and non-pharmacological without bias.

It really would have been wrong not to put pen to paper when there is such a need in this area for alternative ideas and when there is such a shortage of HRT medications in the UK. My insights will hopefully provide that.

Menopause crosses the path of many men on a daily basis including myself. Men will undergo their own hormonal changes also known as Andropause. While men may not experience a change as dramatic as women, I have offered as a man, empathy and compassion during many consultations with females, and this has played a crucial role in supporting them during this transition. In my experience, making you feel heard and understood has gone a long way in helping to resolve certain issues, especially in a sea of uncertainty and where it has been difficult to see a doctor in a timely manner.

There is a good reason why I have written a chapter just for men towards the end of this book. I think it's important for men to help bridge the gap to increase acceptance at both home and in the workplace in his major area of female health. Many of my patients claim that far too many men just brush menopause off without an understanding that this is the second chapter of a woman's life and there is a major upheaval happening, both in and outside of a woman's body.

For balance, a brief section on the male menopause is included as well.

If you're reading this, you're likely somewhere in your 40s or 50s and the winds of change are blowing, signalling the onset of menopause. It's a journey that many women embark on with mixed feelings. But instead of dreading the turbulence, let's explore how to not only accept but also manage this transformative phase of life.

I wish you the very best of luck moving forward.

CHAPTER 1

THE MENOPAUSE ROLLER-COASTER

"Let me introduce myself. I'm Lisa, just a regular woman in her late 40s who was trying her best to keep up with life's challenges. My job in a bustling marketing office kept me on my toes, juggling deadlines, meetings, and many tasks at once. I thought I had it all under control.*

One day though, everything changed. It was one of those moments that catch you off guard, probably one that you or someone you know has experienced. And it couldn't have happened at a worse time.

I was getting ready to give a crucial presentation to my colleagues and some clients. Although I'd done this many times, this particular instance took an unexpected turn. As I started speaking, a strange sensation crept up my neck. My heart raced, and a sheen of sweat broke out on my skin. I attempted to stay focused on my slides, but it was a struggle. The relentless heat just wouldn't let up.

Can you picture it? Standing there, feeling like you're turning into some sort of human lightbulb desperately trying to maintain your composure. It was like my body had chosen that very moment to stage a revolt.

That was the day I had my first hot flush. And as you've got hold of this book, you probably already know it's one of the signs that menopause is around the corner. Trying to escape the awkwardness, I faked a cough, excused myself, and swiftly made my way out, leaving my bewildered colleagues behind.

In the privacy of the bathroom, I peered at my reflection in the mirror, feeling bewildered and more than a little flustered. Fanning myself with my hand, I tried to cool down, asking myself, "Is this what they call a hot flush?"

Back at my desk, things didn't get any easier. Concentration eluded me, and my once reliable memory seemed to be on holiday. During my presentation, my words stumbled, and my thoughts seemed to be on a wild ride.

Despite the understanding nods from my coworkers, I couldn't help but feel a mix of frustration and embarrassment. Menopause had barged into my life unannounced, and I realised that dealing with this new phase of my life would require new understanding of what was going on, a bit of patience and self-kindness"

Lisa's story is not an isolated incident.

Sarah was another woman in her early 50s, juggling a job and a family. As she explained, *"lately, something's was off. One night, I found myself crying for no apparent reason. I had no idea why it's happening, there didn't seem to be any obvious reason"* When Sarah spoke to her co-worker she said that it wasn't her *"it's those hormones playing tricks, they're messing with your emotions."*

Her co-worker hit the nail on the head. Menopausal symptoms can arrive unexpectedly without warning and certainly not by invitation.

"But it's not just tears and mood swings; anxiety creeps in. You could find yourself awake at night, worrying about everything and yet at the same time forgetting stuff like it never existed!"

Let's have a look at of some the aspects of menopause and also rediscover the vibrant, confident, and amazing person you are!

Embracing the Change: East Meets West

Menopause is something you've heard about it in passing, but it always felt like something that happened to others. Until, one day, it happens to you.

It's a natural process pointing towards the ending of a woman's ability to have children. It is a universal experience for women so you are not alone; you are not the first and certainly won't be the last to experience the multitude of changes. During my research into the subject matter, I found attitudes and approaches towards menopause can vary across cultures.

Menopause in the East

According to a Malaysian study, women lack information on the topic and receive less support as they approach menopause. Muslim women did not seek medical attention unless they had serious symptoms since they considered the menopause phase to be a normal occurrence. They also thought that menopause was a normal phenomenon and should be accepted as a symptom of ageing. (Ishak NN et al. 2021)

According to research done in Haryana in India, women welcomed menopause since it freed them from what they felt as cultural pressures and the "polluting" effects of menstruation. Low-income Indian women, whose voices are rarely heard, had a range of menopausal experiences, which were highlighted in the study. (Singh et al. 2020)

Research on menopause in China, Japan, and Korea is limited, but some studies have been conducted on the topic. A study conducted in Hong Kong and southern China found that while, 96% of women from Hong Kong and 73% from southern China had heard of menopause, only 38% and 21%, respectively, could correctly define it. The study also found that women who had a higher level of education and were employed, were more likely to have a positive attitude towards menopause. (Haines et al. 1995)

The Japanese attribute both cultural and biological factors when it comes to menopausal issues. Menopause doesn't appear to be a concern for all Japanese women. The majority of studies tend to emphasise nutrition as the primary factor in Japanese women's lack of symptoms. The good health of these women, according to researchers is "thought to be a result of a combination of diet, exercise, universal public education, equal access to high-quality healthcare, and a long-standing practise of preventative healthcare". (Melby 2005, 2007)

The West

According to available research, women in western countries generally view menopause negatively. (Singh et al. 2002)

This is unfortunate and in contrast to developing countries like India, where menopause is accepted in a more positive light. I know this first-hand because when I visit, I frequently ask my family and related women how they view menopause. Their answers can vary but on the whole, it is widely accepted as part of natural change in female health and in a positive light, and the use of HRT is quite low in society as a whole.

Western medicine has traditionally focused on the biological aspects of menopause. Older women in the West have also been shunned both in the workplace environment and in media in general. It's almost like "well you're too old now and not really fit for purpose anymore", but there is growing recognition of the importance of considering menopause in its broader social and cultural contexts. This has also been highlighted by celebrities and a growing culture of acceptance in this area of health.

Women's experiences of menopause may be influenced by gender norms, familial and sociocultural factors, and how female ageing and the menopausal transition are viewed in their culture (WHO 2022).

It is also worth noting that menopausal symptoms vary considerably by race/ethnicity and are least common among asian races (Green et al. 2009).

With the challenging demographics our planet is facing, the global population of postmenopausal women is growing. Menopausal changes could be viewed as almost acting like a signpost in offering women an important opportunity to reassess their health, lifestyle, and goals moving forward.

Accepting and Embracing This New Phase

Embracing this area of health, which is a natural and inevitable phase of a woman's life, can be challenging but also transformative in its journey. Here are some steps that I think may help you truly embrace and navigate this new chapter in your life:

Acceptance is the foundation of embracing menopause. It's about acknowledging that this natural transition is a part of life's continuous journey. When we look at cultural differences around the world, how you go about viewing this major change in your life can be critical in your ongoing experiences. The change is here now, and for good, so start thinking of this as an opportunity to improve your life rather than as a setback as negative media would portray.

Menopause isn't a sign of weakness, inadequacy, or ageing; it's a testament to your body's resilience and adaptability. Your body is amazing! and it will continue to be so right throughout your life.

"Imagine my surprise when I realised that I was stepping into the world of menopause. I mean, I'd heard about it, sure, but it always felt like something that happened to other people. Until, one day, all the symptoms arrived at my doorstep. Hot flushes, mood swings, you name it! So, I told myself, "Okay, this is happening." I had to stop thinking of it as some sort of curse and start seeing it as just another part of life's journey. It wasn't a sign of weakness or getting old; it was a natural transition."

To truly accept this new chapter of your life, it's best to let go of societal stigmas and expectations. Society isn't suffering, you are! Your personal and professional life should not be dictated by social media and the all-too-common belittling boss. Understand that it's not a personal failure or something to be ashamed of. It's a shared experience among women worldwide.

By embracing acceptance, you free yourself from unnecessary worry and anxiety. Instead of dwelling on what you can't change, you can focus on how to make the most of this new chapter. It's the first step towards finding peace and empowerment during menopause.

Knowledge is indeed power when it comes to menopause. Understanding the physical and emotional changes happening in your body can make this transition less daunting. Taking the time to educate yourself about menopause's various aspects, from hormonal shifts to common symptoms will empower you to take action. I have taken the liberty to add knowledge and awareness as part of the educational component of this book, I hope you will find it useful.

"knowledge became my best friend on this journey. I had to educate myself about what was going on. It' was like driving abroad; you need a map to figure things out.

I started reading up on menopause, the hormonal changes, the typical symptoms, and the possible ways to manage them. Understanding what was happening in my body made me feel less lost and confused. It was like having a torch in the dark. Knowledge gave me a sense of control and confidence"

Knowing what to expect can help you prepare both mentally and emotionally. It allows you to differentiate between typical menopausal symptoms and potentially concerning health issues, providing peace of mind.

Consider reading reputable books, and articles, or consulting healthcare providers who specialise in menopause. A balanced approach empowers you to make informed decisions about your health and well-being.

Chat chat chat and then chat some more! In fact, insist on it. Menopause doesn't need to be a solitary journey. Sharing your experiences and concerns with friends, family, or support groups can provide much-needed emotional support. You'll often find that you're not alone in your feelings or symptoms.

"I remember sitting with my best friend, Sarah, one evening. We were on the wine, and I just blurted out, "You won't believe the hot flushes I've been having!" We laughed about it, and she shared her own experiences"

Opening up about your menopausal journey to a willing ear, can strengthen relationships and create a network of understanding and empathetic individuals who offer comfort during challenging times.

"Talking about it made me realise that I wasn't alone. My friends had stories and tips to share, and we supported each other through the ups and downs"

Moreover, discussing menopause openly reduces the stigma surrounding it. It encourages others to share their experiences and seek help when needed. It's important to break down the barriers that have shrouded this natural phase in silence and misunderstanding.

Self-care is not selfish care. It should be a non-negotiable aspect of embracing menopause. It is a major part of this book and my personal, non-drug mantra.

It encompasses physical, emotional, and mental well-being. Prioritising self-care can significantly improve your quality of life during this transition.

"I knew I had to prioritise physical self-care. So, I started taking daily walks just around the estate, not power walks, just slow, peaceful strolls. I was so relaxed and I knew it was helping my

flushes. I also paid a little more attention to what I ate, I read up about how my bones might be changing so I thought I would include foods that were higher in calcium and vitamin D"

Getting your head around "me" time is crucial here. Far too many women (and men) are wrapped up in work-work balance rather than work-life balance. This book will help you to re-evaluate this. Establish a routine that focuses on a healthy balanced diet, enough sleep, and plenty of movement, for example exercise. Those people who engage in regular physical activity release hormones called endorphins. These make them "feel good" because they help with both mood swings and combat stress.

Adequate sleep is essential, as menopause, often disrupts a restful slumber. Create a calming bedtime routine, free from screens and distractions, to improve sleep quality.

Emotional self-care involves recognising and addressing your feelings. You're likely to experience a wide range of emotions during menopause, and this is perfectly normal. Engage in activities that promote emotional well-being, such as journaling, or mindfulness exercises.

Embracing menopause can also involve a **spiritual dimension**. This does not mean going to church every week or pushing a religious agenda. For many women, this transition is an opportunity for self-reflection, growth, and deepening their spiritual connection. This book's emphasis is on accepting holistic practices.

"Spirituality wasn't something I'd paid much attention to before menopause. But during this journey, it became a source of strength. I started meditating regularly, just a few minutes each day. It was like finding a quiet oasis amid chaos. Meditation helped me connect

with my inner self, and find peace as well as improve my symptoms. I also found solace in nature. I'd take long walks in the park and sit by the pond nearby, I would listen to the ducks and just started feeling a deep sense of connection to the world around me"

Explore your spiritual beliefs and practises during this time. Whether it's meditation, prayer, or spending time in our beautiful English countryside, these practises can provide solace and guidance. They help you connect with your inner self and find strength and resilience.

Spirituality can offer a sense of purpose and meaning; your inner voice helping you navigate the emotional ups and downs of menopause with a sense of serenity.

Self-compassion is a vital aspect of embracing menopause. Instead of criticising yourself for mood swings, memory lapses, or physical changes, give yourself the same consideration and understanding as you would a close friend.

Understand that these changes are part of the natural ageing process. It's not your fault, and you are not alone in experiencing them. The event has happened so beating yourself about won't change it. Self-compassion involves practising self-kindness, common humanity, and mindfulness.

"I had to learn not to be too hard on myself when I had mood swings or forgot where I put my keys (again). This took a little bit of effort but I just reminded myself that I was doing the best I could in a difficult situation.

It was like having a gentle inner voice that said, "Hey, it's okay. You're going through a lot right now, and that's perfectly normal." Being nicer to myself just made me feel more at ease with the ups and downs that were happening"

When you approach menopause with self-compassion, you acknowledge that you are doing the best you can in a challenging situation. This mindset fosters self-acceptance and resilience, allowing you to navigate menopause with grace.

Setting realistic expectations about your body and appearance during menopause is essential. This is always a difficult one to accept when I talk to patients about it.

Menopause may bring about physical changes like weight gain, shifts in skin elasticity, changes in hair texture, etc. Everyone is different and their response to menopausal changes will be different too.

Rather than striving for an unattainable ideal, focus on maintaining overall health and well-being. Look for alternatives that boost your confidence and appearance for example hair supplements that actually work. This is now a new chapter of your life and your health becomes ever more important moving forward. Celebrate the aspects of yourself that remain strong and vibrant. Understand that you are still the same person with the same worth and value, regardless of physical changes.

"I got realistic about what was going on in my body. I understood from what I read that menopause might bring some physical changes, like a few extra kilos or changes in my skin, so I just focused on staying healthy and feeling good and just let nature do its thing. It was kinda weird at first but I began embracing the quirks and imperfections that make us beautifully unique. I think realistic expectations allowed me to be kinder to myself"

Set goals that align with your present self. This realistic approach to self-image can alleviate unnecessary stress and self-criticism.

Menopause marks a transition in your life, and with it comes newfound opportunities. As one door shuts another opens. It doesn't just slam in your face!

"It's like finishing one book and eagerly starting a new one. As my children grew and I reduced my hours at work, I found more time for myself. I embraced this newfound freedom by joining my local painting class, something I tried in my early 20s but had to give up when I got pregnant. It was great to start this up again"

Look upon this time as a chance to explore new hobbies, travel, or pursue long-neglected interests. Whether it's learning a musical instrument, joining a dance class, or taking up painting, engaging in creative and fulfilling activities can boost your sense of self-worth and joy.

This phase can also be an opportunity to strengthen relationships, deepen connections, and explore new horizons in your personal and professional life.

Menopause is a time to **celebrate the wisdom** you've gained over the years. It's a testament to your resilience and the wealth of knowledge and experience you've accumulated. If you have had children, then just remind yourself of how epic a journey you have made, raising a family. It is like being the CEO of your own household, you are the glue that binds everyone. This is something that particularly dawned on me when my mother passed away.

Embrace your wisdom as a source of strength and empowerment. Use your life experiences to make informed decisions about your health, relationships, and overall well-being.

Recognise that you have valuable insights to offer, whether it's mentoring a younger generation, pursuing new career opportunities, or engaging in advocacy or community work. Your wisdom is a gift that continues to grow and enrich your life and it's a gift that keeps on giving!

Staying positive is a biggie! While menopause can bring challenges, it also offers positive aspects. It signifies the end of menstruation, freeing you from the monthly cycle. This newfound freedom can be liberating and open doors to new experiences.

"No more monthly cycles to worry about! It was like a weight lifted off my shoulders"

Menopause can also usher in a sense of confidence and self-assuredness. Many women report feeling more comfortable in their skin and less concerned about societal expectations. View the changes as a natural part of your life's journey and celebrate the possibilities that lie ahead.

There is so much positivity to be discovered at this stage of a woman's life, and keeping this at the forefront of your thoughts as the transition begins will have a significant impact on how you experience menopause.

Seeking support beyond medication is a powerful way to navigate menopause. Whether it's through professional help, menopause support groups, therapy, or talking to friends and family, sharing your feelings and experiences can provide comfort and understanding.

"I was a bit hesitant at first, as I didn't want to come across as a whinger but I was talked into joining a menopause support group, where I met other women on similar journeys. We shared our stories, and just generally chatted about stuff. It felt good actually, we had

a few laughs about our menopausal mishaps. It was like getting to know a small group of people who had experienced what I was going through"

Support groups, in particular, offer a sense of community and camaraderie. They allow you to establish a connection with those walking a similar path, offering mutual encouragement and empathy.

Professional support, such as therapy or counselling, can also be beneficial, especially if you're struggling with mood swings, anxiety, or other emotional challenges. Trained professionals beyond doctors can offer advice and coping mechanisms suited to your circumstances; examples could include Physiotherapists, Yoga practitioners, and Naturopaths. Remember to get your man involved here as well, the more he can help you the better life will be for the both of you. See Chapter for Men.

I tell all the women I speak to, menopause is an investment in yourself. It's like a bank account where you are depositing self care into yourself. You won't see growth initially, but over time the investment will pay off. It is important to see it this way because this next chapter in your life is all about your health and you absolutely matter!

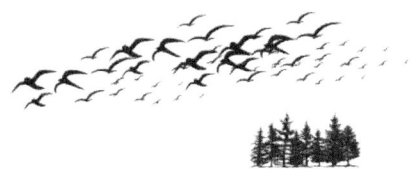

CHAPTER 2

MENOPAUSE UNVEILED:
The Oestrogen Exodus

What is Menopause?

Health definitions will vary depending on which country or health jurisdiction you are based. Organisations and regulators will create their own parameters in which to define the terminology. Disclaimer: The following definitions are broad-based for the average person and may vary from regulatory definitions.

The National Institute of Clinical Excellence in the UK defines menopause as **"a biological stage in a woman's life when menstruation stops permanently due to the loss of ovarian follicular activity. It occurs with the final menstrual period and is usually diagnosed clinically after 12 months of amenorrhoea"** (NICE, 2019). Amenorrhoea is the term doctors use to describe a woman having no periods.

Menopause signposts to a woman that her reproductive years are over and this is signified by her last and final period. It happens to every woman and is a completely natural biological process. It can be viewed as an end to fertility.

It is commonly called "the change" because a woman is changing from a fertile to a non-fertile period in her life. It can occur anywhere from the ages of 45 and 55 but typically appears to be the age of 51, although many women are stopping their periods much earlier which could be defined as premature menopause. (NICE, 2019)

The process of the Menopause is primarily driven by hormonal changes. A woman is born with "X" number of follicles that can turn into eggs in the reproductive years. As a woman ages, her ovaries gradually produce fewer eggs. The ovaries become less responsive to hormones, and there is a decline and fluctuations in the production of two key hormones: Oestrogen and Progesterone.

Hormones are basically just chemical messengers in the body that go around helping cells and organs to function and work in certain ways.

Menopause affects every woman and the symptoms can vary greatly from person to person.

Perimenopause, often referred to as the menopausal transition, is the stage leading up to menopause in a woman's reproductive life. It can be thought of as the time when a woman's body begins to undergo hormonal changes and experiences symptoms that eventually lead to menopause; this is when you start to notice the symptoms. It's like having PMS (premenstrual syndrome) symptoms that gradually get worse.

This phase generally begins in the mid-40s but can be earlier. It's normally about 5-7 years before the menopause.

During perimenopause, the levels of the two key hormones, oestrogen and progesterone start to fluctuate. This can result in a range of physical and emotional changes which vary in intensity and duration. These hormones are the main ones that oversee the woman's sexual and reproductive development. Menstrual periods also fluctuate and can become lighter, shorter, heavier, and longer and in general, unpredictable.

It is also in this phase that the unpleasant symptoms start i.e., hot flushes, night sweats, breast tenderness, and many others. It's important to be aware that while many women experience symptoms during perimenopause, the severity and duration of these symptoms can vary widely from person to person, from months to years until the hormonal storm settles down.

Understanding the natural transition and accompanying changes that occur during perimenopause can help women manage their health and well-being during this phase.

Postmenopause is the part of a woman's life that starts after menopause and continues into old age. It's the phase that begins after she has completed the menopausal transition, which includes perimenopause and menopause itself.

Once a woman has reached the menopausal milestone, she is considered to be post-menopausal after that.

Postmenopause represents a significant and extended period in a woman's life, typically spanning the remainder of her adult life. During this phase, the hormonal changes that occur during peri and menopausal transitions will be in the process of stabilising.

The symptoms experienced during perimenopause, for example hot flushes, may also stabilise in the later part of this phase and in line with hormonal level consistency.

The post-menopausal phase is a completely natural and normal part of a woman's life. You are not the first or last to go through it and it does not signify the end of vitality or productivity. Many women find this phase liberating, as they are no longer burdened by the menstrual cycle and can focus on their health, interests, and personal growth. Regular healthcare check-ups and a healthy lifestyle are essential for maintaining well-being, and longevity, and reducing hospital admissions during the post-menopausal years. I know it can be hard to see a GP these days, but it's important to stay on top of things and have regular milestone tests and check-ups when they are due.

Medically Induced Menopause

This term is also known as surgical menopause or artificial menopause, is a situation in where a woman's menstrual cycles and ovarian function cease abruptly due to medical interventions, such as surgery, or certain medical treatments. Unlike natural menopause, which occurs gradually over several years, medically induced menopause occurs suddenly, and is often accompanied by distinct challenges and considerations.

Causes and Methods of Induction:

Bilateral Oophorectomy: One of the most common causes of premature menopause is where both ovaries are removed in a surgical procedure known as bilateral oophorectomy. This may be performed as a preventive measure in cases of a high risk of ovarian cancer or as part of a hysterectomy (removal of the uterus) for conditions such as uterine fibroids or endometriosis. When both ovaries are removed, the body loses its primary source of oestrogen and progesterone, leading to immediate menopause.

Radiation Therapy: Radiation therapy, commonly used in cancer treatment, can damage the ovaries and disrupt their hormone-producing function. Depending on the type and dosage of radiation, this can result in either temporary or permanent menopause.

Chemotherapy: Certain drugs can harm the ovarian follicles, leading to a condition known as chemotherapy-induced ovarian failure (CIOF). This can result in the temporary cessation of menstruation and the onset of menopausal symptoms during treatment, which may or may not be reversible after treatment ends.

Medication Induced: There are a certain group of medications called gonadotropin-releasing hormone (GnRH) agonists. These are used in the treatment of conditions such as endometriosis, uterine fibroids, and certain cancers. They work by suppressing the production of oestrogen, inducing a state similar to menopause. However, this is usually reversible after stopping the medication.

The symptoms of medically induced menopause can arrive quite suddenly and be more intense compared to normal menopausal symptoms due to the immediate cessation of hormone production. Unfortunately, the abruptness of the transition can make symptoms feel more severe, which may affect a woman's self-esteem and body image.

A surgical process that removes your uterus is called a Hysterectomy. Depending upon the type of hysterectomy performed the ovaries may or may not be left intact. If kept, then it usually doesn't cause immediate menopause. Although periods stop, the ovaries still produce the hormones and release eggs.

Primary Ovarian Insufficiency (POI). This is a medical condition in which a woman's ovaries cease to function properly (also known as premature ovarian failure) before the age of 40. It is characterised by a loss of ovarian function, including a deterioration in the production of the female sex hormones oestrogen and progesterone, which can lead to irregular or absent menstrual periods and, in some cases, infertility. POI is different from natural menopause, which occurs around the age of 50, as it occurs much earlier in a woman's life.

POI can occur without an identifiable cause, but in some cases, it may be associated with underlying medical conditions, genetic factors, autoimmune disorders, or exposure to certain treatments or chemicals.

In these cases, Hormone Replacement Therapy may be recommended to protect vital organ functioning. This will be on top of other support measures such as psychological or fertility options as a diagnosis of POI can have considerable negative effects on a woman's mental and emotional health. It may affect body image, fertility desires, and overall quality of life.

The Menstrual Cycle: Navigating the Hormonal Highway

So, why should you care about hormones and the menstrual cycle during menopause? Because, ladies it's all connected, Your hormones, whether they're taking you on a wild period ride or sending you into a hot flush frenzy, are the secret sauce of your menopausal experience.

Hmm.... so what are hormones? I don't hear you ask!

Well, hormones are basically chemical messengers made by various glands and tissues around the body, for example the pancreas or the thyroid gland. These messengers play an essential role in coordinating various physiological processes throughout the body (for example blood sugar levels or weight), maintaining a stable environment within the body (homeostasis), and influencing growth, development, mood, and overall health.

Hormones travel through the bloodstream to target cells or tissues, where they bind to specific receptors and trigger a response; think of a hormone as a key which then binds/slots into a lock which is the receptor.

When the key turns it has the effect of opening the door, just as when the hormone binds to the receptor it initiates some kind of response.

Each hormone has a unique function, and they work together in complex networks to regulate the body's functions.

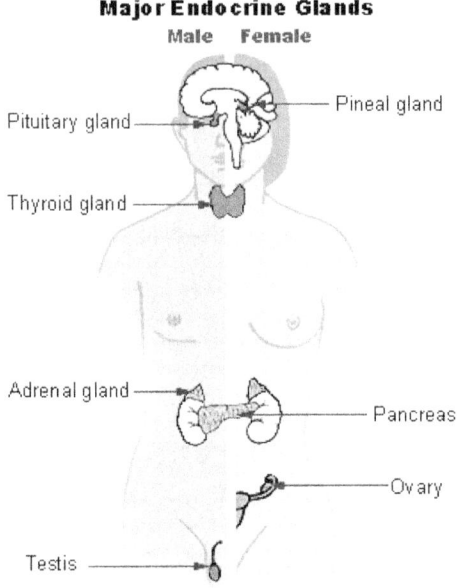

Figure 1: Major Endocrine Glands
https://upload.wikimedia.org/wikipedia/commons/9/9d/Illu_endocrine_system_New.p
ngUS Government, Public domain, via Wikimedia Commons

Pineal Gland: Melatonin (important in sleep)

Pituitary Gland: Follicle stimulating hormone (FSH), Luteinising Hormone involved in egg release, Prolactin (menstrual cycle and milk formation)

Parathyroid Gland: Parathyroid Hormone (PTH) involvement in bone regulation

Thyroid Gland: Thyroxine (T4) and Triiodothyronine (T3) Involvement in weight, metabolism and energy production

Adrenal Gland: Produces a number of hormones including Adrenaline and the Steroid hormones and Cortisol (Fight or Flight and Stress response, Immune system, Sex hormone production)

Pancreas: Insulin and Glucagon (blood sugar regulation)

Ovary: Oestrogen and Progesterone (fertility and menstrual cycle)

Testes: Testosterone (male reproduction and secondary sexual characteristics)

"I ovary-act when I'm on my period. It's not my fault; my hormones are just doing stand-up comedy!" — Unknown

In menopausal women, several key hormones play crucial roles, and their fluctuations are at the heart of menopausal symptoms and changes. Here are the key hormones involved:

Oestrogen is one of the primary female sex hormones in the body. It has many roles as you will see further on including skin elasticity, maintaining strong bones, and the all-important regulation of monthly cycles. Oestrogen levels decline significantly during menopause, leading to a variety of symptoms, including flushes, breast tenderness, and vaginal dryness to name a few.

Progesterone works in conjunction with oestrogen to regulate the menstrual cycle and support pregnancy. Progesterone production decreases during menopause, contributing to menstrual irregularities and other symptoms.

Follicle-stimulating hormone (FSH) helps regulate the menstrual cycle by stimulating follicle development in the ovaries. It is made by the pituitary gland and FSH levels rise significantly as the ovaries become less responsive to its signals during menopause.

Luteinising Hormone (LH), like FSH, is also made by the pituitary gland and its involvement is in the ovulation process. LH levels also increase as the ovaries become less sensitive to its feedback signals during menopause.

Gonadotropin-releasing hormone (GnRH) from the hypothalamus in the brain, regulates the release of FSH and LH. During menopause, the hypothalamus becomes less sensitive to hormonal feedback, leading to fluctuations in GnRH secretion.

Testosterone: Although its effects are predominantly expressed in males, women also produce small amounts of this female hormone, which can influence mood, libido, and energy levels. Testosterone levels may decline during menopause, contributing to changes in sexual desire and overall energy.

Cortisol made by the Adrenal glands that sit like little "hats" on top of your kidneys, helps you cope with stress and maintain a regular sleep-wake cycle. Just like other hormone-producing organs, the adrenal glands can also experience fluctuations during menopause. Stress can have a more pronounced impact on adrenal function, leading to variations in cortisol levels, which can influence mood and energy. (Speroff et al. 2018)

Some women may experience a situation called "adrenal fatigue" or "adrenal exhaustion." While this term isn't recognised as a medical diagnosis, it suggests that prolonged stress during menopause can potentially strain the adrenal glands, leading to fatigue and other symptoms.

"Sarah was a go-getter juggling career, family, and social commitments. But as menopause arrived, her energy levels plummeted. Fatigue, mood swings, and sleep problems took hold. A healthcare check suggested adrenal exhaustion; a consequence of relentless stress"

This wake-up call forced Sarah to prioritise self-care, realising that menopause demands more than inner strength—it requires nurturing your well-being. Sarah's story teaches us that embracing this phase means honouring your body's needs and finding balance amidst change.

It's important to note that hormonal changes during menopause are complex and vary among individuals. I have kept things simple in an attempt to spare you from boredom!

The Menstrual Cycle

Ladies, let's face it – your bodies are like a symphony; your brain is the conductor and hormones are the orchestra. They play a crucial role in everything from energy levels to our emotions. But here's the thing – most of you were never told how this hormonal masterpiece works. You were just handed a box of tampons and told to deal with it. So let's take a quick look.

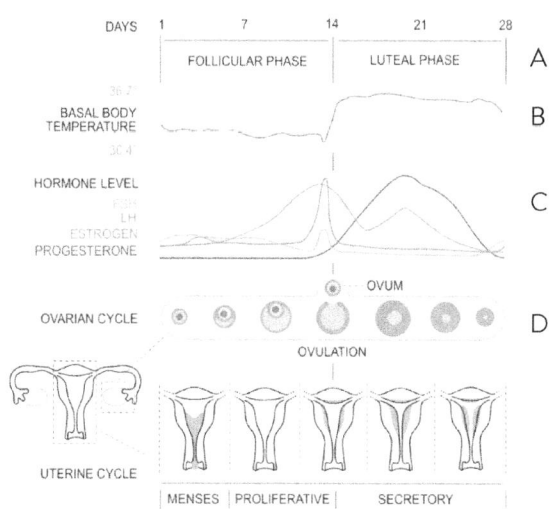

Figure 2 : The menstrual cycle. Stages of the proliferation of the lining of the womb (endometrium)and eventual breakdown and shedding (menstruation) By Isometrik - Own work, CC BY-SA 3.0, https://commons.wikimedia.org/w/index.php?curid=8703107

A= Names of the two phases of the cycle

B= Temperature changes over the cycle

C= Main hormones involved

D= Egg creation and release (Ovulation)

Build up and shedding of the lining

I know what you're thinking, "why on earth has he put this complicated picture up"

"The more that you read, the more things you will know. The more that you learn, the more places you'll go." - Dr. Seuss

A simplified version of the cycle is as follows:

There are **3 phases** in the cycle which involve the monthly release of an egg from the ovary, the thickening of the uterine wall ready for egg implantation, and then the eventual breakdown of it which is termed "menstruation" when the lining is shed.

The Monthly Gathering: Imagine at the beginning of each month you were watching an episode of Britain's Got Talent. The judges in the programme would include the charming LH (Luteinising Hormone), the trusty FSH (Follicle Stimulating Hormone), the vivacious oestrogen, and the no-nonsense progesterone (PG). Their mission? Select the most promising egg and make it shine like a star.

There are **4 main hormones** that interact with each other and keep the cycle running throughout the month. Initially, FSH is a hormone that is released from the pituitary gland and is carried around the body in the bloodstream, and picked up by the ovaries. This phase is called the Follicular Phase.

The Great Egg Audition: Now imagine we are going through each of the competition rounds on the programme. It's getting tough! Each egg from an ovarian chorus line would strut its stuff, hoping to be the chosen one. We have strict hormonal judges and only the egg with the most potential would get the golden ticket to stardom.

Inside the ovaries are hundreds of follicles which contain the immature eggs or ova. FSH causes some of the follicles to grow and mature and one ova matures faster than all of the others. FSH causes the ovaries to start to make and release oestrogen.

The Ovarian Palace: We are now in the finals and the judges are in hot debate. Once the winning egg was selected, the plan would be to move it into a luxurious ovarian palace, where it would be pampered and prepared for its big debut to the world.

Oestrogen, detected by the uterus, starts building up the lining of the womb ready for egg implantation. The rise of oestrogen also feeds back on the pituitary signalling it to stop producing more FSH enabling the release of only 1 mature egg.

The Showstopper Encore– Ovulation: Finally, the moment everyone had been waiting for arrived – ovulation night! As if pomp and ceremony are called to the occasion, the successful egg makes its entrance to the audience including the charming sperm (talent scouts) who can't take their eyes off it!

Oestrogen also stimulates the pituitary to release LH. The rise in LH is detected by the ovaries which triggers the release of a mature egg from the follicle, in other words ovulation, around about mid-month. The remains of the follicle (now called the Corpus Luteum) produce progesterone (PG) which is carried around in the bloodstream.

PG switches off LH production in the pituitary and also continues to inhibit FSH production as well. PG also keeps the uterine thick and supportive of a possible implantation (Luteal Phase).

The After-party – The Luteal Phase: After the Ovulation show, a fabulous after-party is thrown in the uterine theatre. Everyone who had helped put on the performance was invited. It was a chance for the winner to meet the talent scouts to celebrate and prepare for the next cycle.

Once the egg arrives at the uterus it is either fertilised by sperm in which case it embeds into the uterine lining and progesterone is continued to be made by the ovaries which triggers all of the changes of pregnancy.

If the egg is unfertilised the follicle stops producing progesterone and oestrogen, the levels of these hormones fall and the lining of the uterus breaks down and menstruation happens where the egg is also shed in the period. The fall in the level of PG is the trigger for the pituitary to start producing FSH and the cycle repeats.

This is all a bit dramatic but you can see how complex the menstrual cycle can be. The ebb and flow of egg release, and uterine lining shedding (period) repeats monthly and continues into a woman's 40's.

Natural changes that start happening to the cycle are usually an indication that perimenopause has begun. Fluctuations in oestrogen and progesterone mean that feedback loops back to the brain stop working efficiently which then dysregulates the cycle. This can lead to periods being erratic and difficult to predict.

Blood tests can usually confirm hormone levels and doctors can make decisions based on this and other factors that may affect a woman's well-being whether they are in the menopausal arena.

(Guyton et al. 2006, Vander et al. 2001, Tortora et al. 2017).

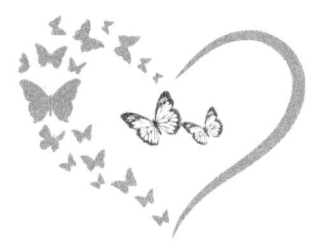

CHAPTER 3

OESTROGEN AND PROGESTERONE:
Hormonal Besties!

"**M**y doctor decided to raise my HRT's oestrogen dose. Whilst I was not happy about his decision, it did give me some relief though. But it had taken me ages to get an appointment and finally be heard. After consulting with HR, I came back to work after having 5 months off, but my hormone difficulties have not been fixed. Although my levels are not perfect, I am still experiencing symptoms, they are not as bad as they were in the past. My boss seemed happy to see me though! Along with making adjustments to my HRT, I've found that changing what I was eating and making other adjustments at home, improved both my physical and emotional well-being, which have somewhat eased my symptoms. Wow, what a palaver!"

Stories like the above are common place everywhere and just go to show how powerful the nature of hormones are, and how they control everything!

Oestrogens, often referred to as the "female hormones," are a diverse group of compounds that play pivotal roles in a woman's body throughout her life. While we often hear about them in the context of reproductive health, their influence extends far beyond that. Let's have a quick look at them, understanding their types, and their critical functions in the body.

Oestrogens are quite the powerhouse here and just like other hormones, their role is vast and complex. They play a crucial role in giving women their unique sex characteristics such as breast development, an hourglass figure with a wide hip-to-waist ratio, and the way fat tends to be distributed around the hips and thighs.

They also have a hand in regulating blood pressure, keeping the menstrual cycle in check, and maintaining energy levels, libido, memory, and mood. In addition, oestrogen is the key bone regulator in both men and women, which is why lower levels put you at a higher risk of developing osteoporosis. Oestrogens are also present in men but in smaller amounts, Testosterone dominates here.

So, you can see why it's such a big deal when levels decline.

Oestrogens are not monolithic; they come in different forms, each with its distinct purpose. Think of them as a versatile ensemble cast, with individual members taking the spotlight at various stages of a woman's life.

Oestrone (E1): As women age and transition into different life stages, Oestrone steps into the limelight. It may not be as potent as oestradiol, but it still plays a crucial role in hormonal equilibrium, even in menopause.

Oestradiol (E2): This is the star of the oestrogen show, known for its potency and prevalence during a woman's reproductive years. It's the most powerful of the three and is responsible for regulating the menstrual cycle and maintaining ovarian health.

Oestriol (E3): It primarily makes its presence felt during pregnancy, contributing to the development of the placenta and supporting foetal growth.

In the realm of female reproductive physiology, menopause stands as a defining chapter, being marked by intricate hormonal changes. Central to this narrative is the reduction of oestrogen levels, specifically oestradiol.

When you need oestrogen replacement therapy, it's usually the synthetic form of oestradiol that your doctor prescribes.

Something to keep in mind is that as women go through menopause, the adrenal glands step up to the plate and take over the task of producing the extra sex hormones, along with other hormones like testosterone, DHEA, and cortisol.

However daily stress and this extra burden on the adrenal glands can sometimes lead to adrenal exhaustion. Although it might not be an official clinical diagnosis, this could be one of the reasons why women experience those typical menopausal symptoms of fatigue general achiness, and weight issues. (Nelson et al. 2001, Soules et al. 2001, Richards 1980, Burger 1999).

"I'm not tired, I'm just taking a break from being fabulous!" – Unknown

Typical Menopausal Symptoms

Depending on where you source the information, It's been reported that there are some 50 plus symptoms of the menopause; here are the most common ones experienced:

Skin: Hot Flushes, Night Sweats
Thin, itchy, very dry skin, pimples/acne or whiskers, loss of elasticity and collagen
Hair loss, electric shocks, tingling, numbness and crawling.

Weight Gain
Bloating as if you were having a period
Sore/swollen breasts

Central Nervous System: Migraine, Mood swings, anxiety, depression, and socially withdrawn
Uncontrolled emotions e.g. crying or sobbing
Anger and shortness of temper, brain fog and memory issues, indecisiveness
Poor sleep quality and insomnia
Tiredness to exhaustion

Heart palpitations, cardiovascular and osteoporosis Issues

Join stiffness, aches and pains

Irregular uterine bleeding which can vary from light to heavy
Bladder issues
Vaginal dryness and discharge
Painful sex and loss of libido
Recurrent infections and blood in urine

Because there is a complex interplay between many hormones beyond oestrogen, it's likely that if you are experiencing any of the above symptoms in your 40s and it's ongoing, you may be experiencing the change.

"At 46 years of age I was depressed, had trouble sleeping, my body ached, and also my anxiety started to get worse. When I saw the doctor he reckoned I was too young to be going through menopause. I asked to be tested for it though. When he said no, I didn't need it, I was pretty upset at how dismissive he was, so I got it done privately. When the results came back it showed that my levels of oestrogen were quite low. So, had I left it to my arrogant GP, I would still have not known. It just goes to show you have to put your foot down. I alone knew my body. I changed my doctor and was put on HRT"

Perimenopause Diagnosis

When you do a pregnancy test with a kit you buy from the pharmacy, it is dependent on hormone detection in the urine. The test looks for a hormone called human chorionic gonadotrophin (hCG). This is usually made in the body when you are pregnant and starts showing up in the urine approximately 6 days after fertilisation. Most tests claim a 99% accuracy rate and kits are sold widely throughout the UK.

But when it comes to menopause, things are not so simple. The symptoms can vary widely among women, making it difficult to establish a clear-cut diagnosis based solely on them. Then you have unreliable fluctuations in hormones, including outliers such as testosterone. Cultural taboos and women feeling awkward initiating conversations with their doctors also add to the mix of an accurate diagnosis. Finally, there is variability in the age of onset which makes it difficult to predict when an individual woman will experience menopause.

The National Institute of Clinical Excellence (NICE) guidelines (2019) in the UK recommends diagnosis based on symptoms and irregular periods. No lab tests, no imaging either. They also state;

"Consider using an FSH test to diagnose menopause only:

- in women aged 40 to 45 years with menopausal symptoms, including a change in their menstrual cycle
- in women aged under 40 years in whom menopause is suspected (see also recommendations on diagnosing and managing premature ovarian insufficiency)"

Please note these guidelines are under review.

Now your doctor may want to do other tests for example a thyroid check in case the symptoms are a manifestation of some other issue going on in the body, and not menopausal.

This is a discussion for you and your doctor as you're going to need a personalised approach to your health issues.

Progesterone

Progesterone emerges as a quiet yet essential player. It tends to be overshadowed by its better-known counterpart, Oestrogen, however, this hormone wields significant influence over a woman's body throughout her life.

The types include:

Natural Progesterone (P4): This is the hormone produced by the Corpus Luteum, which, mentioned earlier in the menstrual cycle, is the remainder of the shell of the released egg during the menstrual cycle. It acts like a temporary hormone-releasing structure formed in the ovaries after ovulation. Natural progesterone plays a fundamental role in maintaining a healthy menstrual cycle and preparing the uterine lining for potential egg implantation.

Synthetic Progestins: These are synthetic compounds designed to mimic the actions of natural progesterone. They are commonly found in contraceptives, hormone replacement therapies, and treatments for certain gynaecological conditions.

Progesterone takes centre stage in the second half of the menstrual cycle, post-ovulation. It prepares the uterine lining for potential embryo implantation, maintaining the uterine environment for a healthy pregnancy. During pregnancy, progesterone plays a pivotal role in maintaining the uterine environment, preventing premature contractions, and supporting foetal development.

The hormone also has a calming effect on the central nervous system. It can alleviate symptoms of anxiety and promote a sense of tranquillity and well-being.

Maintaining Bone Density: Of course, hormones rarely work by themselves in isolation. Progesterone contributes to bone health by stimulating bone formation and reducing the risk of osteoporosis.

Testosterone in Women

As if things weren't complicated enough along comes testosterone which, to say the least, has been subject to controversy over the years. This female hormone has been associated with masculinity which has meant it has largely gone unrecognised in its role in women.

Of all the male-associated hormones or Androgens, testosterone is the most dominant. The body works like a symphony, no one hormone works in isolation to achieve a specific outcome; they all work together. For example, you hear about insulin all the time in blood glucose regulation but you hear very little about glucagon. This hormone has the opposite effect of insulin. Both are involved in keeping our blood glucose levels steady, it's just that it's far more nuanced than you think and you don't hear about it as much. This is very similar in the case of testosterone.

This androgen is involved in libido, muscle mass and strength, fat distribution, and psychological well-being. In the UK it is being recognised as having a role alongside HRT medication and so women are flocking to have testosterone levels tested as well as their other hormones. Testosterone levels may be taken into account when your doctor is discussing your health issues with you.

The Hormonal Duet

Oestrogen-Progesterone Balance: In the premenopausal years, oestrogen and progesterone engage in a delicate dance, maintaining the menstrual cycle's rhythm. However, as menopause approaches, oestrogen levels decline more dramatically than progesterone, altering this balance.

"Before the pandemic, my periods were fairly predictable, but now? I have been absent for an entire month. Normally, I don't have painful periods, but the one I had in January was really awful. It was also unpredictable; it would vanish entirely for a few days before coming back. And Feb? Nope, nothing at all. I can't be pregnant. The nurse checked for that a few days ago when I had a routine checkup. God I miss being regular, hopefully, fingers crossed this month"

Fluctuations and Symptoms: During perimenopause, the transitional phase leading to menopause, progesterone levels may fluctuate. This can lead to menstrual irregularities, including heavy or irregular periods, and potentially contribute to mood swings and sleep disturbances.

Following menopause, progesterone production significantly decreases, as the ovaries stop releasing eggs. With oestrogen levels on the decline, progesterone's role becomes less prominent. However, there is always a fine balance in the control of bodily hormones, and where the decline of progesterone is far greater than oestrogen it leads to a situation called Oestrogen Dominance.

This hormonal imbalance is often associated with conditions such as endometriosis, polycystic ovary syndrome (PCOS), and certain cancers. (Cleary et al. 2009)

It can be common in the early stages of the menopause transition and can occur years before menopause.

Oestrogen dominance in menopausal women can occur due for several reasons. One disruption occurs when oestrogen remains at its regular level, but progesterone levels begin to drop, leading to a relative excess of oestrogen.

Another imbalance can result when extra oestrogen is added to the system through diet, and lifestyle choices that influence how oestrogen is metabolised and energy is regulated. (https://www.womenshealthnetwork.com/hormonal-imbalance/estrogen-levels-estrogen-dominance/)

Certain health conditions, such as obesity and stress, can also lead to oestrogen dominance. Obesity can result in higher oestrogen levels because fat tissue in a postmenopausal obese woman makes oestrogen. Stress increases cortisol levels, which can deplete progesterone levels, affecting the oestrogen balance. (Cleary et al. 2009)

Symptoms of oestrogen dominance can vary between individuals and depend largely on the severity of the hormone imbalance. However, common symptoms often associated with high oestrogen levels in women include decreased sex drive, increased premenstrual syndrome (PMS) symptoms, irregular periods, mood changes, difficulty concentrating, bloating, hot flushes, breast tenderness, weight gain, and insomnia.

(https://www.letsgetchecked.com/articles/estrogen-dominance-symptoms-and-signs/)

Treatment for oestrogen dominance often involves addressing the underlying causes and restoring hormonal balance. This can include changes in lifestyle, such as improving diet and reducing stress, as well as medical interventions like hormone replacement therapy.

As menopause unfolds, the hormonal landscape evolves and changes on a very individual basis. While this transition can bring challenges such as altered periods, mood swings, and disruption of sleep, it also signifies a new phase of life, ripe with opportunities for growth and self-discovery.

"Jenny, a woman in her early 50s, found herself at the crossroads of menopause. Now her journey through this transformative phase was not without its challenges, but it also became a path of self-discovery.

During a particularly sleepless night, Jenny decided to do something different. Instead of tossing and turning in frustration, she grabbed a notebook and began to write. It started with simple journal entries, documenting her symptoms and daily experiences. But as the days turned into weeks, something remarkable began to happen.

Writing became Jenny's sanctuary, a safe space where she could express her thoughts and feelings without judgement. It was as if the ink on the pages held the power to release the pent-up emotions she had kept hidden for so long. She wrote about her fears, her insecurities, and her hopes for the future.

She started to recognise patterns in her mood swings and learned to anticipate the onset of hot flushes. She discovered the therapeutic benefits of mindfulness and meditation, practices that helped her regain a sense of calm amidst the hormonal storm.

Through support groups and conversations with friends who were also navigating menopause, Jenny realised that she was not alone in her struggles. Sharing her experiences and hearing the stories of others reinforced a sense of community and friendship that had been missing from her life"

Hormone Replacement Therapy (HRT): Balancing the Scales of Menopause

The journey through menopause, characterised by hormonal shifts and a range of associated symptoms, can be a challenging one for many women. For decades, Hormone Replacement Therapy (HRT) has been a significant player in the menopausal landscape, offering relief from distressing symptoms and improving the quality of life for countless women.

Hormone Replacement Therapy, often abbreviated as HRT, emerged as a groundbreaking approach to alleviate menopausal symptoms.

The use of hormone replacement therapy (HRT) dates back to the 1960s and peaked in popularity in the 1990s. In the USA, the first HRT and chronic postmenopausal diseases clinical trials got underway in the late 1990s.

The primary goal of HRT is to replace the hormones—namely oestrogen and progesterone—that the body's ovaries no longer produce in sufficient quantities during menopause.

Types of Hormone Replacement Therapy

Oestrogen-only HRT: This form of therapy is typically prescribed to women who have had their uterus removed (hysterectomy). It provides oestrogen alone, helping alleviate symptoms like hot flushes, night sweats, and vaginal dryness.

Combined HRT: In cases where the uterus is intact, a combination of oestrogen and progesterone or synthetic progestin is prescribed. This combination helps protect the uterine lining and reduce the risk of endometrial cancer.

Cyclical HRT: Where a combination approach is used for women who are showing menopausal symptoms but still have their periods. This is where oestrogen is taken daily but progesterone is only taken on the last 10-14 days of the month or 3 months.

For more information on HRT please visit the NHS website which explains in greater detail. The link can be found at https://www.nhs.uk/medicines/hormone-replacement-therapy-hrt/

Benefits of Hormone Replacement Therapy

Relief from Menopausal Symptoms: HRT is highly effective in alleviating the main hallmark symptoms of menopause, including hot flushes, night sweats, mood swings, and vaginal dryness. However, please be aware HRT is not going to be a cure-all for symptom relief.

Improved Bone Health: Oestrogen plays a crucial role in maintaining bone density. HRT can help reduce the risk of osteoporosis and fractures in post-menopausal women.

Cardiovascular Benefits: Some studies suggest that HRT may have protective effects on the cardiovascular system, reducing the risk of heart disease.

Vaginal Health: HRT can alleviate vaginal dryness and discomfort, improving overall vaginal health and sexual well-being.(Gartlehner et al. 2022)

Risks and Considerations

Improvements in HRT have come a long way since its inception. Although HRT offers significant benefits, it's essential to be aware of potential risks no matter how low and make informed decisions in consultation with a healthcare provider:

Breast cancer: HRT has been associated with an increased risk of breast cancer, particularly when used for more than five years.

Ovarian cancer: HRT has been associated with an increased risk of ovarian cancer.

Endometrial hyperplasia and carcinoma: Oestrogen-only HRT has been associated with an overgrowth of the lining of the uterus (hyperplasia) which potentially leads to carcinoma (cancer). Adding progesterone to oestrogen therapy can reduce this risk. This is why HRT comes in a combined pack with 2 types of pills/products one containing oestrogen, the other progesterone.

Cardiovascular disease: HRT has been associated with an increased risk of heart disease, stroke, and blood clots.

Gallbladder disease: HRT has been associated with an increased risk of gallbladder disease.

Dementia: HRT has been associated with an increased risk of dementia in women over the age of 65, however, this is inconclusive and is an ongoing area of research; the results of which may well change in the future.

Urinary incontinence: HRT has been associated with an increased risk of urinary incontinence.

(Hodis et al. 2022, Breast Cancer. Org 2023, Cancer Research UK 2023, Pourhadi et al. 2023)

They type of HRT used by clinicians will vary depending on your age, circumstances and risk factors. Gels and patches have a better side effect profile than tablets. Whatever method of HRT is chosen, please remember you may need to get together with your doctor to experiment with what type and dosing suits you best, and also remember that it can take up to 3 months for the full effects of HRT to be known.

"I had heard great things about hormone replacement treatment (HRT) from co-workers and acquaintances, and I was quite eager to give it a try. But the doctors I met discouraged me because I was at high risk for breast cancer because my mother had the disease. But I thought this wasn't the case because she didn't develop it until

later on in life. I was told that older women tend to be more susceptible"

The Evolving Landscape: Recent Research and Findings

Over the years, HRT has been the subject of extensive research, and recent findings have shed light on its benefits and risks. Healthcare providers increasingly emphasise personalised HRT plans, considering a woman's unique medical history, risk factors, and preferences.

Low-Dose Therapy: Lower-dose HRT regimens are explored to minimise potential risks while maintaining symptom relief. In my humble opinion, this would be the way to go, combining a dose of HRT alongside practices mentioned in this book with the intention of either lowering HRT dosing to find a minimum effective dose as relief is obtained, or completely coming off HRT with the supervision of your health provider if you are deemed clinically unfit to have it. Remember you always have a choice.

Bio-identical Hormones: Some women opt for bio-identical hormones, which are identical in terms of molecules to those naturally produced in the body. Research on their safety and efficacy is ongoing. This is a controversial area.

Bio-identical hormones are man-made and are designed to mimic the hormones made by the body's glands. Bio-identical hormone replacement therapy (BHRT) can help people who suffer from a hormonal imbalance or who might not make enough hormones naturally.

BHRT can help reduce some of the symptoms of menopause such as hot flushes, night sweats, and vaginal dryness. It can also improve sexual experience, improve mood, and decrease symptoms of menopause.

However, the term bio-identical hormone does not have a standardised definition and can mean natural, compounded, plant-derived, or chemically identical to the human hormone structure. Compounded bio-identical hormone replacement therapy (cBHRT) is custom-made in special pharmacies and doesn't come under the same scrutiny as regulated hormone replacement therapy (HRT).

BHRT has been shown to improve skin elasticity, strengthen bones, keep romance alive, and reduce discomfort during sex. However, the benefits and risks of BHRT can vary depending on the individual, and the duration of treatment should not be more than a few years. (Zilberstein 2023, Newson et al. 2109, Files et al. 2019)

It is important to talk to your healthcare provider to get to the root of the underlying hormonal imbalance and map out a personalised treatment plan.

Because the area is unregulated in the UK, BHRT is not recommended by either The National Institute for Health and Care Excellence (NICE) or the British Menopausal Society.

Non-hormonal approaches, such as cognitive-behavioural therapy, herbal supplements, and lifestyle modifications, are gaining attention as viable options for symptom management. These are the foundations of this book and the online programme found at **www.sisstas.com**

An understanding of the pros and cons of HRT is crucial. It's essential to engage in open and informed discussions with your doctor or healthcare providers, weighing individual health factors and preferences. While HRT continues to be a valuable tool for many women seeking relief from menopausal symptoms, it's just one piece of the puzzle. A holistic approach to menopausal health includes maintaining a healthy lifestyle, incorporating regular exercise, managing stress, and fostering a supportive network of friends and family.

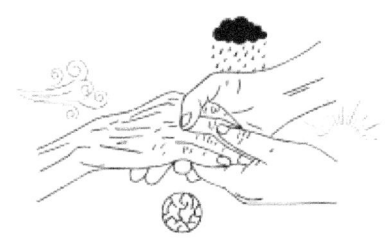

CHAPTER 4

EPIDERMAL EPIPHANIES:
Your Skin's Journey

Hormones play a starring role in the menopausal skin saga. Oestrogen, which gradually declines during menopause, has a profound influence on skin health. It's responsible for maintaining elasticity, moisture, and thickness. As oestrogen levels decrease, the skin's relationship with moisture undergoes a dramatic shift.

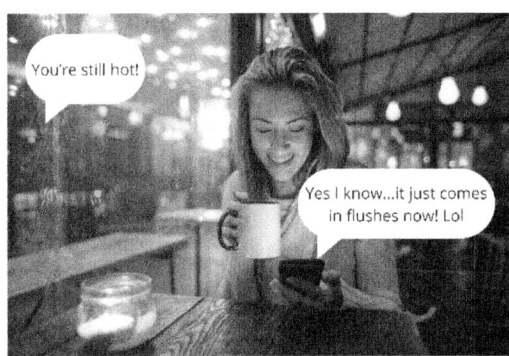

Figure 3: Modified Photo by Andrea Piacquadio https://www.pexels.com/@olly/

Simplified Section of the skin

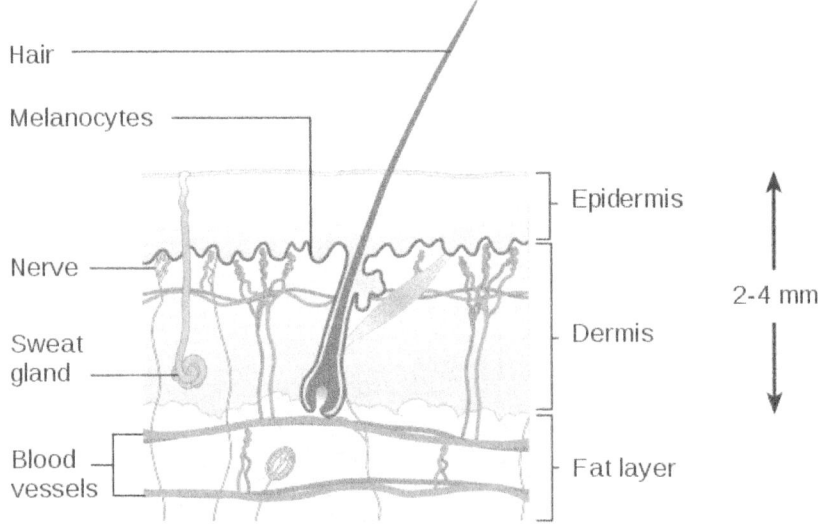

Figure 4: Simplified section of the skin.
Diagram_showing_the_structure_of_the_skin_CRUK_371.svg
Cancer Research UK, CC BY-SA 4.0 <https://creativecommons.org/licenses/by-sa/4.0>, via Wikimedia Commons

Oestrogen is almost like a guardian angel for the skin. Amongst many other things, It helps stimulate the production of hyaluronic acid, (that beauty buzzword that is everywhere!) a substance that acts as a natural moisturiser, holding water in the its cells.

With oestrogen's decline, the skin loses its ability to retain moisture efficiently. As a result, menopausal women often experience increased dryness, flakiness, and a dull complexion

Oestrogens significantly affect skin physiology, targeting certain cells called keratinocytes, fibroblasts, melanocytes, hair follicles, and sebaceous glands. Each of those cells will have a different function.

Oestrogen insufficiency decreases the defence against damage caused by oxidation (particles that involve oxygen leading to damage and ageing); skin becomes thinner with less collagen. The reduced elasticity due to the loss of collagen leads to increased wrinkling, increased dryness, and reduced permeation of blood vessels. The skin loses its protective function; the ageing process is associated with hair loss, changes in pigmentation, skin cancer, and wound healing. Other symptoms reported include acne, pins and needles, and skin "crawling". (Thornton 2013)

"I used to take my skin for granted. It was the one thing I didn't have to worry much about. Sure, I had my skincare routine, but it was more about pampering myself than addressing any real concerns. I felt confident in my skin.

But then menopause came, and my skin seemed to lose its will to live. It's like my complexion decided to rewrite the rules.

At first was the dryness. My once-supple skin suddenly felt parched and tight. It was as if all the moisture had evaporated overnight. No matter how much moisturiser I slathered on, it was a never-ending battle to keep my skin hydrated.

Then came the blemishes. Acne, at my age? I couldn't believe it. I thought I had gotten rid of pimples back in my teens, but why were they making a comeback now? It was frustrating, to say the least

I read stories on Facebook support groups and I realised that I wasn't alone in this struggle. Many women like me were facing similar skin-related challenges during menopause. It wasn't just about vanity; it was about feeling comfortable in our skin and maintaining our self-confidence.

So, I decided to go on a mission to understand my changing skin better. I read up on the science behind these transformations and sought advice from a dermatologist"

You can see now how a multi-billion dollar industry exists just for skincare!

Several other factors contribute to the dryness and ageing observed during this life stage:

Decreased Sebum Production: Sebum is the skin's natural oil, and it's vital for maintaining hydration. As women age, their sebum production tends to decrease as well.

Sun Damage Accumulation: Over the years, sun exposure can take a toll on the skin, and its effects become more apparent during menopause. The accumulated damage from UV rays can lead to the formation of age spots, uneven tone, and a loss of radiance.

Lifestyle Factors: Smoking, poor nutrition, lack of exercise, and excessive alcohol consumption can all exacerbate skin ageing. Menopausal women who engage in these habits may experience more pronounced changes.

As circulating hormones decline due to natural ageing or disease, so does the robustness of the natural skin as a barrier.

Oestrogen helps to prevent the ageing process by thickening the skin and increasing the collagen content whilst also strengthening the epidermal barrier.

(Quatresooz 2007)

There are 2 main types of oestrogen receptors in the skin and they have control over the dermal layer. Over time lack of oestrogen and other androgen hormones affect not only the structure of the skin but also other functions such as wound healing, the sebaceous gland, and differentiation and hair growth. (Makrantonaki 2009)

Anti Ageing Strategies

There are several strategies women can employ during menopause and combat dryness and ageing:

1. Hydration is Key
Invest in a high-quality moisturiser and use it regularly, (you get what you pay for these days, check reviews before you buy) Look for products that contain hyaluronic acid or ceramides, which can help retain moisture. I'm sure you already know this but using a moisturiser on your face, jawline, and neck every day can help keep the skin hydrated and reduce the appearance of fine lines and wrinkles. Drink plenty of water over the day and avoid the dehydrating effect of frequent hot baths or showers. You would be surprised at how fuller your skin looks through adequate hydration; beauty comes from within!

After cleansing, apply moisturiser immediately while your skin is still moist, as this will help lock in extra moisture.

2. Sun Protection Matters
The sun is particularly damaging to the skin and is a huge contributor to the ageing process. This is through oxidation and free radicals creation (unstable molecules that can cause disease and ageing) which damages the skin itself.

Always wear sunscreen with broad-spectrum protection, even on cloudy days and even in countries like the UK where the sun doesn't come out that often. A wide-brimmed hat and sunglasses can offer additional defence against UV rays. Sunscreen should be used every day to prevent age spots and other signs of sun-damaged skin. Check that the product you are buying has some sort of Sun Protection Factor (SPF) rating or something to say about protecting against UV light damage.

3. Cleansing Routine

Your skin comes with its natural oils, so choose a gentle cleanser that won't remove those oils. Exfoliating products that shed dead cells can help make the skin appear brighter in tone and more youthful looking. Toners can also help with the cleaning process removing dirt and bacteria which may not be possible with warm water alone. Toners will also have different effects depending on your skin type, for example, alcohol-based toners will only dry out further, dry skin. It's better to seek expert advice on matching a product with your skin type for maximum benefit.

4. Healthy Lifestyle Choices

Prioritise a balanced diet rich in antioxidants, vitamins, and minerals. Stay hydrated by drinking plenty of water. Engage in regular exercise, and consider quitting, or at least reducing smoking/alcohol if applicable. A vital component is sleep and stress both of which have an impact on outward appearance. The key here is consistency, quitting smoking for a day for example is going to have minimum impact on your skin compared to quitting forever.

5. Skincare Ingredients

There are 2 types of agents that can make a significant difference in anti-ageing products. Antioxidants and Cell Regulators.

Antioxidants including Vitamin B3 (niacinamide), C, and E are the best because of their ability to penetrate the skin to the inner layers due to their small size. Once there they have anti-inflammatory, anti-proliferative properties as well as maintain humidity, increase Collagen 1 and 3, and have photo-protective abilities. (Ganceviciene et al.2102)

Another compound showing a lot of promise is Astaxanthin (ASX). This has been shown to have photo-protective, antioxidant, and anti-inflammatory effects.

Because of its unique structure, ASX seems to have the ability to mop up highly damaging particles that lead to the ageing process (called free radicals), reducing chronic inflammation and skin damage. The best quality is from marine algae rather than the mass-produced version from the petrochemical industry. (Davinelli et al. 2018)

The other group which are cell regulators stimulates the production of collagen and elastic fibres. Examples here are retinol, retinaldehyde, tretoin, polypeptides, and botanicals.

Look for the ingredients on the label. Consult with a dermatologist or skin specialist for personalised recommendations.

6. Low dose HRT
Medication in combination with the above will help restore some of the issues regarding the skin. Post-menopausal women taking HRT may have higher levels of ceramides (basically fats that make up the epidermis) that help retain moisture. Keep in mind though that the dose should be effective at it's low therapeutic level.
(Farage, M. A., & Miller, K. W. 2009)

Hot Flushes and Night Sweats

"At 54-year-old I was working in a busy department store where I would sort of float about but be typically be in the women's shoe section.

Around about six months before making an appointment with my doctor, I first experienced hot flushes. I was experiencing them during the day and I hadn't a period in 14 months. Thankfully, I was not having night sweats, but my hot flushes during the day were becoming stronger and more regular.

Due to my flushes, I struggled more and more at work. I also had to wear this awful uniform, I wasn't sure of the fabric mix but it really didn't agree with me or my skin. Drinks weren't allowed on the shop floor, and it was difficult to constantly run to the bathroom.

I would dread the onset of a hot flush as I could feel the sweat dripping down my back. I just felt hot and uncomfortable and highly embarrassed in front of customers – not to mention my colleagues and my male boss"

What causes the hot flush?

It is not 100% known why hot flushes occur. It has been suggested that during menopause, the body's thermostat in the brain called the hypothalamus, becomes more sensitive to slight changes in body temperature.

In other words, there appears to be an imbalance in core body temperature between the two zones of sweating (upper), and shivering (lower) thresholds in what is called the thermoregulatory zone.

This means that the body tends to overreact to slight fluctuations in body temperature and the physical response then becomes exaggerated. This wouldn't be the case if you were not menopausal.

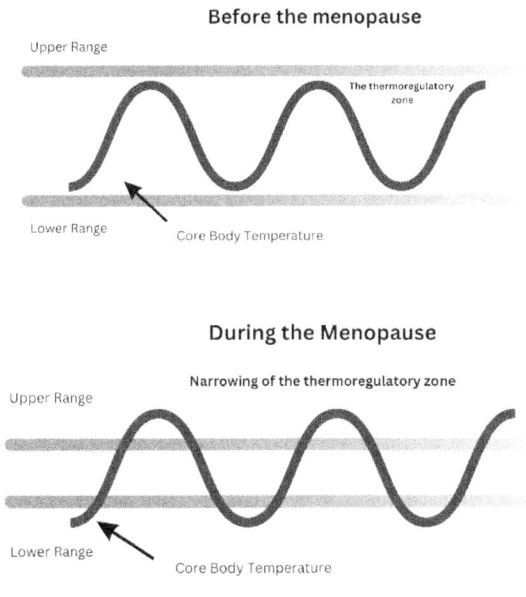

Fig 5: Hot flush illustration

The hormonal orchestra within the hypothalamus plays a significant role in defining the thermoregulatory zone's boundaries. During menopause, hormonal shifts, primarily the decline in oestrogen levels, influence the hypothalamus's sensitivity to temperature fluctuations (Santoro, N., & Randolph, J. F. 2011)

Oestrogen, known for its wide-reaching effects, regulates the release of chemicals released by nerve endings (neurotransmitters) involved in thermoregulation.

The decline in oestrogen levels affects the way neurotransmitters behave. Of particular interest are Noradrenaline (Norepinephrine) and Serotonin (the happy hormone).

Noradrenaline, responsible for triggering vasoconstriction (which is a squeezing of blood vessels), can become overactive in response to temperature changes. This overactivity leads to rapid and intense vasoconstriction, causing hot flushes. (Bansal R, Aggarwal 2019)

Serotonin, another key player, also experiences fluctuations during menopause, contributing to changes in thermoregulation. (Freedman 2005)

Progesterone, the other hormone to oestrogen has a calming effect on the central nervous system, potentially counterbalancing some of the excitatory effects of oestrogen withdrawal. (Genazzani et al. 2003)

The brain receives signals from various sensors (like mini thermometers) throughout the body, including those in the skin and the organs. These sensors send information about bodily temperature changes to the hypothalamus, which then interprets the signals and decides whether to start the cooling or heating mechanisms. (Cannon (1929)

I have overly simplified this highly complex area as there are other hormones and chemicals involved here.

The overall result is a hot flush which is a vasomotor symptom (i.e., due to dilation and constriction of blood vessels) that arrives suddenly as a feeling of heat in the upper body, (face, neck, and chest areas) and begins to extend downward as well as upward. The uneven flushing of the skin is followed by sweating, increased heart rate, and the associated anxiety as you well know. A night sweat is just flushing through the night.

"Jackie, a woman in her early fifties, was sailing through life until menopause brought unexpected turbulence. Hot flushes, night sweats, and anxiety disrupted her once-peaceful existence.

Restless nights left her fatigued, while daytime anxiety attacks hindered her work and strained her relationships. Jackie needed a lifeline.

One day, while scrolling through a menopause support group online, Jackie found hope in the form of Cognitive Behavioural Therapy (CBT). Desperate for relief, she thought she would try it out.

She connected with a CBT therapist and together, they identified her triggers for anxiety and hot flushes.

CBT, she learned, reshapes thought patterns and behaviours, focusing on understanding and responding differently to emotions. They began dissecting her anxious thoughts.

Jackie realised her worries were often irrational. She feared public embarrassment due to hot flushes and constantly worried about having one during meetings or social gatherings, exacerbating her anxiety.

With her therapist's guidance, Jackie challenged these negative beliefs. She acquired relaxation techniques and coping strategies, integrating deep breathing exercises and mindfulness into her daily routine.

Gradually, Jackie noticed changes. Her hot flushes became less frequent and less intense, and she managed her anxiety better.

One afternoon Jackie attended a work meeting without the usual jitters and didn't experience a single hot flush. It was a small victory that marked a significant step toward regaining control of her life.

CBT wasn't a quick fix for Jackie, but it was transformative. It empowered her to rewrite her relationship with menopausal symptoms, shifting from victim to conqueror"

Jackie's story showcases CBT's impact on women navigating menopause's emotional roller-coaster. It equips them with tools to face challenges head-on, emerging stronger, more confident, and in control.

We will be tackling hot flushes and night sweats using CBT later on in the Action component of this book.

Although hot flushes generally last only a few minutes you may be more prone to them if you are overweight, a smoker and drink alcohol. Hot food or drinks, warm environments, and stress can also act as triggers. (Nelson et al. 2005)

"There is some racial and ethnic variation of hot flushes with Caucasian women reporting the highest prevalence and Japanese and Chinese women reporting the least". (Gold et al. 2006)

As hormones fluctuate during menopause so does the signalling to the brain and other areas which affects bodily temperature. These symptoms also known as Vasomotor symptoms can be varied throughout the day and between individuals.

Medications

Here is a list of common medications that have been reported to cause hot flushes(not exhaustive):

Hormonal therapies: Hormonal therapies such as tamoxifen, raloxifene, and leuprolide can cause hot flushes.

Antidepressants: Certain antidepressants, such as selective serotonin reuptake inhibitors (SSRIs) and serotonin-norepinephrine reuptake inhibitors (SNRIs), can cause hot flushes. Examples include venlafaxine, paroxetine, citalopram, escitalopram, and fluoxetine. In contradiction though it has been found that low doses of Venlafaxine and Paroxetine may actually relieve flushes and improve symptoms.

Blood pressure medications, such as calcium channel blockers, and hydralazine.

Chemotherapy drugs: Used to treat cancer.

Steroids: High doses of steroids can affect hormone balance and cause hot flushes.

Opioids: Opioids used for pain relief, such as morphine and oxycodone.

Erectile dysfunction medications: Erectile dysfunction medications such as sildenafil, tadalafil, and vardenafil can cause hot flushes. These have other uses such as hypertension and ulceration on the digits.

Medications that may alleviate Hot Flushes

Hormonal therapies: HRT such as oestrogen and progesterone can alleviate hot flushes. Hormone treatments come in a variety of formulations including creams or gels, patches, implants, rings, and traditional pills.

Antidepressants: As mentioned above certain antidepressants, such as selective serotonin reuptake inhibitors (SSRIs) and serotonin-norepinephrine reuptake inhibitors (SNRIs), can alleviate hot flushes. Examples include venlafaxine, paroxetine, and fluoxetine in low doses. A common issue is that women complain their doctor has put them on anti-depressants and yet they are not depressed! Now you know why.

Blood pressure medications such as clonidine.

Certain anti-seizure medications, such as gabapentin and pregabalin, can alleviate hot flushes.

Fezolinetant: A new drug that is a hormone-free option for treating menopause hot flushes. It works by blocking a pathway in the brain that helps regulate body temperature. This may well be licensed in the UK and other countries by the time this book is published.

The medications mentioned above do not form an exhaustive list. New medications are coming out all the time so always check with your pharmacist for up-to-date information.

Strategies for managing hot flushes and night sweats will be explored in the Action section of this book.

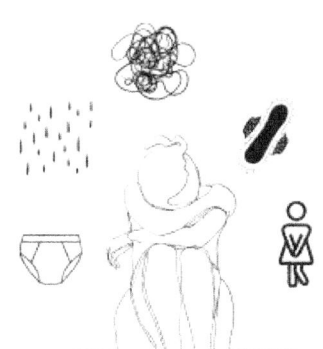

CHAPTER 5

DRY SPELLS, LEAKY MOMENTS:
Genito-Urinary (GU) Symptoms

"One afternoon, I met up with friends for coffee. As we chatted, I discreetly shifted in my seat, trying to find a more comfortable position. I couldn't ignore the subtle discomfort that had been bothering me lately. It felt like my bladder had decided to play tricks on me, and it always happened at the most inconvenient times.

It started innocuously enough. I'd occasionally feel a sudden and urgent need to use the bathroom, but on this particular day, things were different.

As my friends chatted away, I felt a strong demand from my bladder. It wasn't just an urge anymore; it was like a command. I excused myself from the table and hurried to the bathroom, hoping there wouldn't be a queue.

In that moment of privacy, I couldn't help but reflect on how these genito-urinary problems had become a part of my life. I mean how are other women coping with this. This is hideous, It wasn't just the urgency; there was also a persistent feeling of dryness and discomfort, making intimate moments with my partner much harder than it should be"

Genito-urinary symptoms are a part of the menopausal landscape, but they don't have to define a woman's journey. With understanding, support, and a bit of resourcefulness, women can navigate this aspect of menopause and continue to embrace life's adventures with confidence and resilience.

As women age, they may experience a variety of genital symptoms related to menopause. These include dryness, burning, and irritation in the area, sexual symptoms such as lack of lubrication, discomfort or pain, and impaired function, and urinary symptoms such as incontinence issues, recurrent urinary tract infections including blood in the urine and pain on urination.

"These symptoms seem to be directly associated with the lower amounts of oestrogen during menopause. The GU region has oestrogen receptors, and although their amounts decrease with menopause, they can be replenished by taking more oestrogen therapy". (Nappi RE, Palacios S 2014)

When Oestrogen level are high, as seen during puberty and pregnancy, the vaginal micro-environment is preserved by stimulating the maturation and proliferation of the cells that line the vagina and the accumulation of a carbohydrate called glycogen (a form of stored glucose). Ph balance is therefore maintained with the help of bacteria that use the glycogen and also the vaginal lining itself. This acts as both a physical and chemical barrier to external bacteria and other pathogens.

With declining Oestrogens this fine balance is lost which leads to women experiencing various problem in this area.(Amabebe E, Anumba DOC. 2018)

"Additionally, these fluctuations cause the vagina to become less elastic, elevate the pH of the vagina, which alters the flora inside, decrease lubrication, and make the vagina more susceptible to physical damage and irritation, such as painful sex".(Nappi RE, Palacios S.2014)

"A few years back, the dryness started, making it excruciatingly unpleasant to use tampons and engage in sexual activity. My anxiety increased, and my libido plummeted. Due to my underlying issues, I had pleaded with my doctors to prescribe hormone replacement therapy and I eventually got my wish in December and received Ovestin cream a month earlier.

At the age of 47, I wish someone had paid attention sooner. I really had a battle with my GP as i have diabetes and high blood pressure, as doctors are too afraid to touch you for fear of being sued"

Pelvic floor exercises may help with bladder leakage and in general, a woman's sex life. This is explored in the Action Section of the course. Please also see this section on advice for Vaginal Dryness and Pain.

Overactive Bladder and Incontinence

Recent statistics show that women are twice as likely as men to experience urinary incontinence. Research suggests that about 20-30% of young women, 30-40% of women in their middle years, and up to 50% of women in their senior years have this problem.(Kołodyńska et al. 2019)

The main reason behind incontinence is not fully understood, because the problem can affect men and women of all ages and can be due to many changes in the human body and not just the menopause for women. Amongst treatments like surgery, physiotherapy can be significantly beneficial to help control bladder leakage. (Syan R, Brucker BM. 2016)

As mentioned previously a receptor is basically a protein molecule either inside a cell or on its surface which receives a signal or chemical that lets the cell do something in response. Think of it like a lock i.e., the receptor and a key i.e., the chemical which then opens the door i.e.,. cellular response.

Oestrogen receptors are proteins located inside cells that specifically bind to the oestrogen hormone. These receptors are found in various tissues throughout the reproductive and genitourinary tract, including the uterus, vagina, urethra, and bladder.

"I was very upset when I discovered I was unexpectedly wetting myself; it was a nightmare.

I tried drinking less, but this caused headaches and dehydration.

I had heard that bladder weakness could have resulted from childbirth. I discovered though stretched and weakened muscles could be worked back to full strength. So I began a habit of frequently pausing to pee in the bathroom and practising internal clenching which definitely helped but i was changing as sanitary towel roughly four times every day; it wasn't great.

My anxiety shot through the roof to the point that I stopped going out with friends as I felt very embarrassed and paranoid about my pee coming through my clothes. It was awful and made me feel distant. I finally saw my doctor.

I read on a few forums that you could get specific pads for pee that are leak-proof and odour-proof. I tried a few brands before settling on Tena pads. This seemed to be the best. At least i found some relief to the problem"

Simplified Image of Pelvic Floor

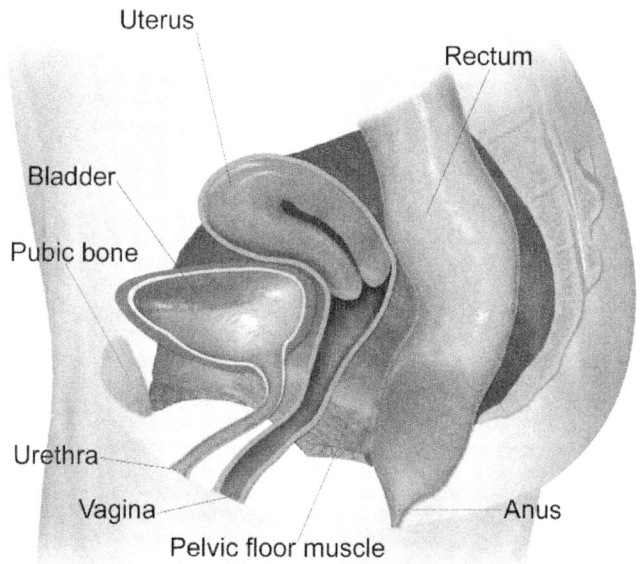

Figure 6:Simplified Image of Pelvic Floor
https://upload.wikimedia.org/wikipedia/commons/3/3f/Pelvic_Muscles_%28Female_Side%29_%28cropped%29.png BruceBlaus, CC BY-SA 4.0
<https://creativecommons.org/licenses/by-sa/4.0>, via Wikimedia Commons

Let's look at the 4 main areas affected.

In the Uterus: As covered previously, oestrogen receptors in the uterus help regulate the growth and maintenance of the uterine lining during the menstrual cycle. As oestrogen levels decline during menopause, the uterine lining becomes thinner and less responsive, leading to irregular bleeding or the cessation of menstruation.

In the Vagina: Oestrogen receptors in the vaginal tissue help maintain the health and function of the vaginal lining. Oestrogen promotes the production of vaginal secretions and the maintenance of the vaginal pH, elasticity, and thickness. As levels decrease, vaginal tissue becomes thinner, drier, less elastic, and more prone to inflammation. This can result in symptoms such as vaginal dryness, itching, discomfort during intercourse, and an increased risk of vaginal infections.

In the Urethra: If we look at the female pelvic area, the little tube that carries urine from the bladder out of the body is called the Urethra. Oestrogen helps keep the urethral tissue healthy, maintaining its strength and elasticity. As levels decline, the urethral tissue can become thinner, weaker, and less capable of maintaining continence. This can contribute to urinary incontinence and the feeling of an infection when you don't have one. With time, the surrounding pelvic muscles may also deteriorate, a condition known as "pelvic relaxation."

In the Bladder: Oestrogen receptors are also present in the bladder tissue. Oestrogen helps maintain the health and function of the bladder, supporting its muscle tone and the integrity of the lining. With decreased oestrogen levels, the bladder tissue may become more susceptible to inflammation and irritation, leading to urinary urgency, frequency, and overactive bladder symptoms.

Of course, other hormones and chemicals will be involved, but I have just focused on the main hormone oestrogen causing these changes so you get an idea of what is happening.

(Santoro, N., et al. (2016), Dennerstein, L., et al. (2010), Drake, M. J., et al. (2017).

Types of Incontinence

Urinary Incontinence has been described by the International Continence Society (ICS) as an "involuntary uncontrolled leakage of urine" due to the bladder not functioning properly.

The main types include:

Stress incontinence is a type of urinary incontinence that causes urine to leak out when the bladder is under pressure.

It occurs when the muscles and other tissues that support the urethra (pelvic floor muscles) and the muscles that control the release of urine (urinary sphincter) weaken.

This weakening can be caused by a variety of factors, including pregnancy and vaginal delivery, pelvic prolapse, nerve or tissue damage in the pelvic area, and ageing.

The main symptom of stress incontinence is leaking urine when you are physically active, during coughing, sneezing, or exercise.

It presents with urinary complaints of frequency, urgency, and pain or burning sensations. Kegel exercises (which we will see later) can help strengthen the muscles that support the urethra. In severe cases, surgery may be considered.

Urge incontinence ("overactive bladder"), due to abnormal bladder contractions. The most common symptom is the frequent and sudden urge to urinate, with occasional leakage of urine.

This can be due to a variety of factors such as bladder inflammation, bladder stones, infection, brain or nerve problems, nerve injury, and prostate conditions.

Treatment for urge incontinence may include treatments such as pelvic muscle exercises, medication, electrical stimulation, or Botox injections.

"So a friend of a friend told me about Kegel exercises just in passing. I didn't give it much thought until it was mentioned again by the GP when I asked her about the bladder issues I had been having. So I tried it, I was desperate to try anything at this point.

I began my Kegel exercise routine, which involved contracting and relaxing the pelvic floor muscles. It was a bit strange at first; it felt like learning to flex a muscle I'd never paid much attention to. But I was pretty determined to have some sort of control over my bladder just to feel less embarrassed.

After a few months, I noticed subtle changes. The urge to rush to the bathroom became less frequent, even my occasional leaks seemed to occur less often. It was quite empowering and I think it boosted my confidence as I just felt so much better about things"

"Believe you can and you're halfway there." - Theodore Roosevelt

Like with most of the issues surrounding menopause, It's important to take action. If you do nothing then nothing changes. If you are suffering then please don't live in the suffering. If you are unsure about what to do then go and seek help. Support extends beyond your GP. It is worth the time and investment to see someone like a Physical Therapist who will guide you accurately on your issues.

We will explore strategies to help with Incontinence further in the Action section of the book.

CHAPTER 6

OSTEOPOROSIS:
Battling a Silent Thief

eet Alice, a vibrant woman in her early 60s who loves life's adventures. She's trekked through the mountains, danced under starry skies, and laughed her way through countless family gatherings. Alice has always been active, vivacious, and full of energy. But recently, she noticed a change – a subtle shift in the rhythm of her life. It started with a sudden twinge in her back while gardening, then a small fracture in her wrist from an innocuous fall. She brushed it off as the inevitable consequences of ageing, but deep down, she knew something wasn't right. That something was osteoporosis, a condition she had heard about but never thought would become a part of her story.

Osteoporosis, sneaks into lives like Alice, robbing them of bone density and strength without warning. It's a condition that affects millions of people, particularly women, as they journey through the years of menopause and beyond.

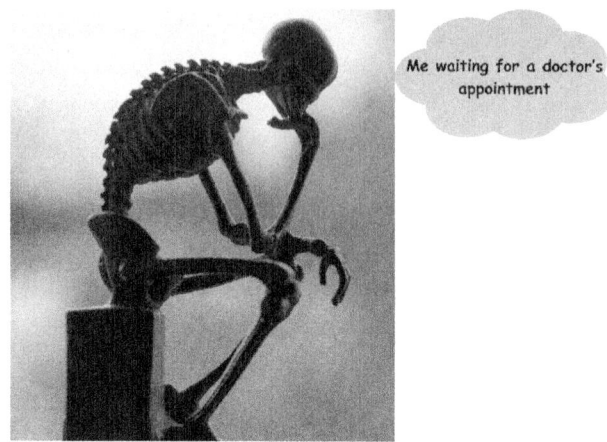

Figure 8: Photo https://www.pexels.com/@adrian-schmidt-56315239/

Reduced bone density and thinning

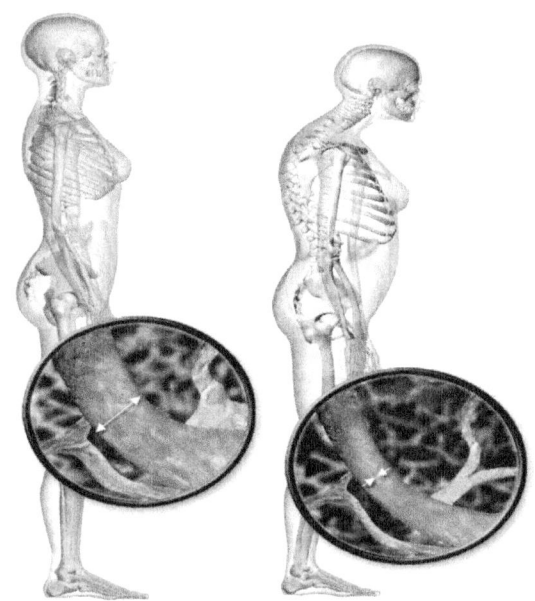

Figure 9: Photo
https://upload.wikimedia.org/wikipedia/commons/d/da/
Blausen_0686_Osteoporosis_01.png
BruceBlaus.Blausen.com staff (2014). "Medical gallery of Blausen Medical 2014".
WikiJournal of Medicine 1 (2). DOI:10.15347/wjm/2014.010. ISSN 2002-4436., CC BY
3.0 <https://creativecommons.org/licenses/by/3.0>, via Wikimedia Commons

Osteoporosis is a "silent disease", a bit like blood pressure that creeps up with the ageing process. It is basically where the body's ability to create new bone doesn't keep up with the loss of old bone.

Oestrogen is a key regulator of bone metabolism in both men and women, but other hormones such as testosterone are also involved to preserve muscle mass and tendons and ligaments. These hormonal changes increase the risk of fractures.

Typical symptoms are:

Stooped posture overtime
Bone pain or tenderness
Rounding of the back also known as "kyphosis"
Height loss overtime

"Given how much cheese i used to shovel away, I suppose I was startled when I was given an osteoporosis diagnosis in 2013.

I was one of the fortunate people whose osteoporosis was only discovered through a regular bone density scan that my family doctor had requested because neither parent had the disease. When I was originally diagnosed, I didn't know much about how it was treated or how well treatments worked. I was started on tablets in hospital, I forget the name now but my GP put me on Prolia when i came home. I was cautious doing things at home like twisting and going up and down the stairs.

So i started some yoga. My diet had to change as well. I make a conscious effort to get my calcium from food sources rather than pills. The doctor told me I should take in 1200 milligrams of calcium every day. Together with 2000 units of vitamin D, I wanted to obtain that as well from food sources. I think younger people should be made more aware of the importance of bone health as well, and getting tests done early"

Osteoporosis

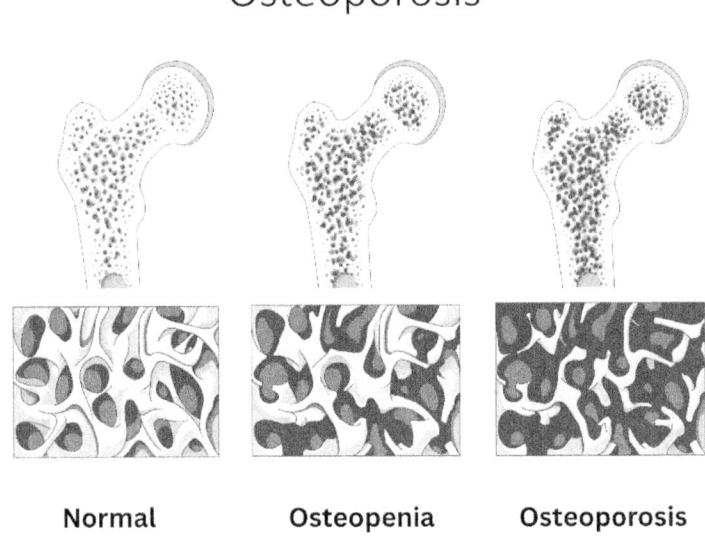

Normal   **Osteopenia**   **Osteoporosis**

Figure 10: Osteoporosis
By Laboratoires Servier - Smart Servier website: Images related to Osteoporosis, Bone structure and Bones -- Download in Power-point format.Flickr: Images related to Osteoporosis, Bone structure and Bones (in French)., CC BY-SA 3.0, https://commons.wikimedia.org/w/index.php?curid=82640910

The loss of oestrogen is associated with declines in bone mineral density. This leads to osteopenia (low bone density), which is a softening of bone. Osteopenia is a pre-cursor of osteoporosis which is the more serious condition where bones have become more porous and brittle.

So why all the bone drama?

The human skeleton is constantly being broken down and recreated and this is known as remodelling.

This involves the removal of old mineralised bone by cells called osteoclasts, followed by the formation of the new bone matrix via cells called, osteoblasts and the new matrix subsequently becomes mineralised. (Minerals are those elements found on the earth and in foods that our bodies need to develop and function normally for example Calcium, Magnesium, and Zinc).

Osteocytes lie within the bone matrix, they respond to mechanical strain and help regulate the creation and mineralisation of bone. Bone remodelling is needed to meet changes in the skeleton through daily wear and tear. It's needed to help repair micro-damages in the bone matrix, prevent the accumulation of old bone, and play an important role in maintaining blood calcium levels. There are a number of hormones that work both locally and throughout the body to maintain bone integrity. (Hadjidakis DJ, Androulakis II. 2006)

In osteoporosis, there is an imbalance between bone remodelling and resorption. The overall result is a loss of bone material and minerals, and a decrease in bone density which makes bone susceptible to fracture.

Osteoporosis risk increases with age and it is estimated that one in three women in the UK will have a fracture in their lifetime based on Osteoporosis.
(https://patient.info/doctor/osteoporosis-pro)

Oestrogen has direct effects on the cells which affect the bone remodelling and resorption process, and so a decline has a detrimental effect on bone stability.

The rate of bone loss is most rapid in the years immediately following menopause and then slows down. Bone mass can be a good predictor of how strong your bones are, and this can be measured using Bone Mineral Density or BMD. A scale has been developed by the World Health Organisation which categorises BMD and is given a value called a T score.

Doctors use this score and other factors to determine fracture risk and to determine what treatment should be used moving forward. The T-score on a bone density report shows how your current bone mass, differs from that of an average healthy adult. The test is called a DXA test or dexa.

The minus values indicate a greater risk of fracture:

Between -1 and +1 is regarded as normal bone density
Between -1 and -2.5 is regarded as low bone density (Osteopenia)
From -2.5 and lower is regarded as Osteoporosis
From -2.5 and lower plus one or more fractures is regarded as Established or Severe Osteoporosis

If you're 50 and older with a broken bone, ask your doctor or healthcare provider whether you need a bone density test.

Breaking a bone is often the first sign of osteoporosis or a patient may notice that he or she is getting shorter or their upper back is curving forward. If you are experiencing height loss or your spine is curving, be sure to consult your doctor or healthcare professional. (Tu et al. 2018)

Risk factors for osteoporosis include ageing, race, body weight, and certain medicines. Women are four times more likely to get osteoporosis than men because of a decrease in oestrogen after menopause.

The older you are, the greater your risk of osteoporosis. Your bones become thinner and weaker as you age. Small, thin-boned women are at greater risk. Caucasian and Asian women are at highest risk. African American and Hispanic women have a lower but significant risk.

Fracture risk may be due, in part, to heredity. People whose parents have a history of fractures also seem to have reduced bone mass and may be at risk for fractures.

Abnormal absence of menstrual periods (amenorrhoea), low oestrogen level (menopause), and low testosterone level in men can bring on osteoporosis.

Anorexia Nervosa is an eating disorder that is characterised by an irrational fear of weight gain; this increases your risk for osteoporosis. A lifetime diet low in calcium and vitamin D makes you more prone to bone loss. (Sözen et al.2017)

Long-term use of certain medications, such as glucocorticoid steroids, some anticonvulsants, and acid blockers can lead to loss of bone density. Check with your pharmacist here to see if any medications you are on put you at risk of lower bone density.

Janine was diagnosed with severe osteoporosis at the age of 49. *"I was devastated when my doctor told me I had extremely low bone density, with a T-score of -4.8T in my spine, according to the DEXA scan. I mean I never saw this coming, what can I do now? I was in shock for a while and thankfully both my husband and my doctor helped me pick up the pieces"*

Treatment Options

Despite the high prevalence of osteoporosis, there are treatment options available.

The goals of managing osteoporosis are to decrease pain, prevent fractures, and minimise further bone loss. For postmenopausal osteoporosis in women, medicines can maintain bone health. Rehab programs can help regain bone health.

Bisphosphonate drugs are usually the first choice for osteoporosis treatment (depending on your jurisdiction). These include alendronate, risedronate, zoledronic acid.

Unrelated to bisphosphonates, another drug denosumab might be used in people who can't take a bisphosphonate, such as some people with reduced kidney function.

Bisphosphonate medications work by reducing the rate at which your bones break down. There are others though that work by speeding up the bone-building process.

Either mechanism strengthens bone and reduces your risk of fractures. Bone-building drugs include teriparatide and abaloparatide.

These bone-building drugs can be taken for only one or two years, and the benefits begin disappearing quickly after you stop. To protect the bone that's been built up, you'll need to start taking a bone-stabilising medication such as a bisphosphonate.

While there are many pharmacological treatments available for osteoporosis, non-drug methods of treating osteoporosis are also available. These non-drug methods aim to slow down or stop the bone loss that leads to breaks. Certain natural remedies and lifestyle changes may help to prevent osteoporosis from developing or slow down the progression of the condition.

Don't rely entirely on medication as the only treatment for your osteoporosis.

An adequate intake of calcium, vitamin D3, and K2 is also required as it helps to reduce age-related bone loss. High sources of calcium are to be found in dairy products, such as milk and cheese. Vitamin D3 and vitamin K2 ensure that calcium is absorbed easily and reaches the bone mass.

As calcium and vitamin D3 recommendations will vary depending on which jurisdiction you are reading this book from, I have not mentioned values here. However, some recommendations can be found here at the Bone Health and Osteoporosis Foundation. (https://www.bonehealthandosteoporosis.org/patients/treatment/calciumvitamin-d/)

Exercise is one of the most effective non-drug methods in the treatment of osteoporosis. It makes bones stronger and helps to maintain healthy bone mass. Weight-bearing exercises, such as walking, jogging, and dancing, are particularly effective in building bone density. Resistance exercises, such as weightlifting, can also help to build bone density.

Exercise can also improve balance and coordination, which can reduce the risk of falls and fractures. The American Geriatrics Society recommends exercising three times a week at a moderate to high intensity, doing weight-bearing exercises, and doing balance exercises to reduce falls and fractures. (https://www.healthinaging.org/a-z-topic/osteoporosis/care-treatment)

However certain exercises may increase the risk of fractures if your bones are already weak.

Remember to always consult with the relevant health professionals such as your doctor, osteopath, physical therapist, and exercise trainer as recommendations will vary depending on your circumstances especially if you are sedentary and have not exercised before.

Quitting smoking and drinking

Smoking and excessive alcohol consumption can increase the risk of osteoporosis. Smoking can reduce bone density and increase the risk of fractures, while excessive alcohol consumption can interfere with the body's ability to absorb calcium. Quitting smoking and reducing alcohol consumption can help to prevent osteoporosis and reduce the risk of fractures.

Low-Intensity Vibration Therapy has also been showing promising results although this type of therapy isn't cheap, however, it is an option. (Rajapakse et al. 2021)

"Since I have a hectic life, maintaining my health and fitness is vital to me. According to a DXA bone scan, I have osteoporosis. My ability to appropriately manage my bone health is being aided by information from the Royal Osteoporosis Society. My pharmacist who is vegetarian suggested I try Flaxseed from the Whole Food Shop and increasing my fibre intake. He said it can be used to aid with the constipating side effects of the painkillers I am taking. I found attending a support group allowed me to meet others going through a similar experience as I am. It makes exercising more fun together"

Falls interventions

Falls are a major cause of fractures in people with osteoporosis. Falls interventions, such as removing tripping hazards from the home, installing grab bars in the bathroom, and improving lighting, can reduce the risk of falls and fractures. Physical therapy can also help to improve balance and coordination, reducing the risk of falls and fractures.

Don't wait for your GP to fix the issue, it may be too late by then. Check online for sources or organisations that are pertinent to your needs.

Alternative therapies

Alternative therapies, such as acupuncture, Tai Chi, and the supplement Melatonin, have been suggested as potential treatments for osteoporosis. While more scientific research is needed on the subject, some herbs and supplements are believed to reduce or potentially stop the bone loss caused by osteoporosis.

Red Clover is thought to contain oestrogen-like compounds. Since natural oestrogen can help protect bone, some alternative care practitioners may recommend its use to treat osteoporosis. However, there's no scientific evidence to show that red clover is effective in slowing down bone loss. (https://www.healthline.com/health/osteoporosis-alternative-treatments)

Surgery

In severe cases of osteoporosis, surgery may be necessary to repair fractures or correct spinal deformities. Your doctor should be able to give you more guidance, or if you cannot get through, try your local pharmacies. They may be able to signpost you to various sources of trusted help.

Osteoporosis and its prevention is a long-term strategy and so won't be covered here in this boot-camp-style self-help book to help manage the more immediate, distressing symptoms of menopause.

Menopausal Joint Pain: Creaking the Code

"In February 2006, when I was 48 years old, I had my last period. I've been experiencing discomfort in all of my joints, particularly, for more than two months. I was working in a small two-story Solicitor's office in Hackney.

Gosh, I had to climb those stairs every day, up and down with all those files. I was confused as to why it was only happening during the day as I was okay in the evening.

Up and down, up and down all day long. It was agony to the point I had to see my doctor as I thought I had arthritis like my mother did. She quickly put me on HRT which helped quite a lot and painkillers which gave me constipation and nausea.

I tried Yoga and stretching for the pain which was so helpful, I just felt so flexible and it allowed me to reduce my dose on all my medications. Looking back now I didn't realise I was perimenopausal then"

Menopausal joint pain can be a silent but persistent hurdle for women, affecting their quality of life and limiting their activities. While it may not be as openly discussed as hot flushes or mood swings, it's a very real part of the menopausal experience.

Pain can take many different forms, and may feel like a dull ache, a twinge, or a shooting sensation. Joints may also feel stiff. While joints themselves are most commonly affected, the pain may also seem to emanate from tendons, muscles, or bones.

These symptoms vary a great deal from person to person, and each individual's experience will be unique. Menopausal joint pain often starts out worse in the morning and gets better as the day's activities loosen up the joints.

Most women complain of back pain, neck pain, as well as pain in the jaw, shoulders, and elbows. Wrists and fingers can also be affected. The pain can be accompanied by stiffness, swelling, or even shooting pain travelling down the back, arms, and legs. Some women report more of a burning sensation, especially after a workout. (Lu et al. 2020)

Why do we get the pain?

To understand joint pain, we need to understand inflammation.

Inflammation is just a natural response by your body's immune system to protect and heal damaged tissues; imagine cutting yourself. So it's like a body's defence mechanism against harmful substances or injury. When an area of your body becomes damaged or infected, your immune system mounts a response by sending inflammatory cells and chemicals to that area. These cells produce a reaction to remove bacteria and other harmful substances and send clotting factors to begin repairing damaged tissue.

You may experience pain, heat, swelling, or redness in the area but eventually, the inflammatory response leads to healing of that injured part.

Inflammation comes in two varieties:

Acute inflammation: The body's reaction to an injury that occurs suddenly, like cutting your finger or a sore throat, etc.

Chronic inflammation: Even when there is no threat from the outside world, your body keeps releasing inflammatory cells mounting a response towards healthy tissue.

Examples of this could include arthritis and respiratory disease.

In Arthritis, Inflammatory cells and chemicals attack the joint tissues, causing an intermittent inflammation that can seriously harm joints and result in pain and deformity.

During menopause, oestrogen plays an important role in maintaining the health of your joints. When levels decline, it can affect the cells within your joints, leading to pain and discomfort.

Within your joints, there are specialised cells called chondrocytes that help maintain the cartilage, which acts as a cushion between your bones. Oestrogen interacts with these chondrocytes, and when levels drop, it can disrupt the normal functioning of these cells.

This disruption can result in the breakdown of cartilage and make your joints more susceptible to pain and inflammation.

There is another type of cell in your joints, called synovial cells, and these can also be affected by changes in oestrogen levels. These cells produce a fluid called synovial fluid that lubricates your joints and keeps them healthy.

When oestrogen levels fall, these synovial cells may become more inflamed and produce more substances that cause pain and swelling in your joints.

Additionally, oestrogen has an impact on your immune system, which plays a role in regulating inflammation in your body. When levels decline, it can disrupt the balance between pro-inflammatory and anti-inflammatory responses, leading to increased inflammation in your joints and contributing to joint pain.

Other factors that can contribute to joint pain during menopause include carrying excess weight, leading a sedentary lifestyle, loss of muscle mass through ageing which leads to joint destabilisation, dehydration, poor diet, smoking, and stress. (Goldring, M. B., & Otero, M. 2011, Hørslev-Petersen, K. 2008)

"My experience with the menopause is not as unusual as I believed it to be for years. Strangely I've never experienced a hot flush like most women. I guess the menopause affects different women in different ways.

I did recall though having pain in my fingers and my left knee which used to wake me up in the middle of the night. This eventually spread to both knees and my hips. I was in agony and sometimes unable to move, sit, or stand.

My GP at the time didn't know and brushed me off with painkillers, eventually, he sent me to see a few specialists and consultants in the hospital. I had tests done including those for Fibromyalgia and Lyme Disease to name a few, but the results came back normal.

So I tried HRT out of desperation, but it didn't seem to help much. I got lucky though, the person who seemed to be most helpful was my physiotherapist, he seemed to think it was menopause and gave me exercises and stretching to do. It definitely helped and with the painkillers and CBD oil, life became more bearable"

Please see the Action section of the book to help with Joint Pain.

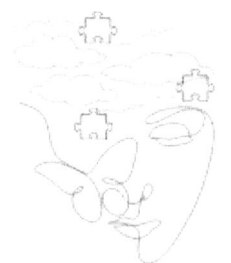

CHAPTER 7

CLOUDY WITH A CHANCE OF WISDOM:
Menopausal Brain Fog

"**M**y peri-menopausal symptoms, including achy elbows, some sleep issues, and a few night sweats, started when I was about 48. I think compared to most women I have read about, I have managed to get through the menopause fairly lightly.

However I think the worst of the issues started just after 48, when I started to feel like my brain was made out of a sieve, I knew very little about menopause and its effects. I began to worry that I might have Alzheimer's disease when I started to lose words.

My kids used to say to me "mum I've told you like three times already"; It was very disconcerting. On the whole, i was better at remembering faces than names, but one day, I couldn't remember my sister's name for a second, and later, I could not recall my former teacher's name either.

I would also forget stuff my husband expected me to know, he thought it was odd and that I should see the doctor. I did panic a bit because my grandfather had Alzheimer's and I know it can run in families"

As we grow older we tend not to be as sharp as we were in our younger days. Menopausal women tend to report brain fog, forgetfulness, and general memory lapses. These women describe the experience as like having a brain made of "cotton wool!"

This is due to the hormonal imbalances happening during this challenging period in women's lives. As Oestrogen has receptors in the brain, a decline in hormones in general will lead to a decline in cognitive function.

Oestrogen has been suggested to be involved in brain nerve health and higher cognitive functions. It appears it also has a protective role from nerve injury caused by toxins, excitatory chemicals, and oxidative stress (which is a type of chemical reaction that can lead to cell damage and ageing).

Nerves are like very fine electrical cables that transmit signals throughout the body. This allows us to do the simplest thing like touching or the most incredibly complex things like thinking. They use chemical messengers called neurotransmitters, these carry messages from one nerve cell to another or a gland or organ.

Oestrogen influences several chemical messengers used by the nervous system to transmit messages between nerves, or from nerves to muscles. Examples of these chemical messengers include acetylcholine, serotonin, noradrenaline, and glutamate.

The nerves that use the chemical Acetylcholine are specifically affected in the memory processes and Alzheimer's disease.

Testosterone and progesterone also work directly with the nerve cells in the brain, affecting mood, memory, and cognitive function. (Henderson 2008, Hidalgo-Lopez et al. 2020)

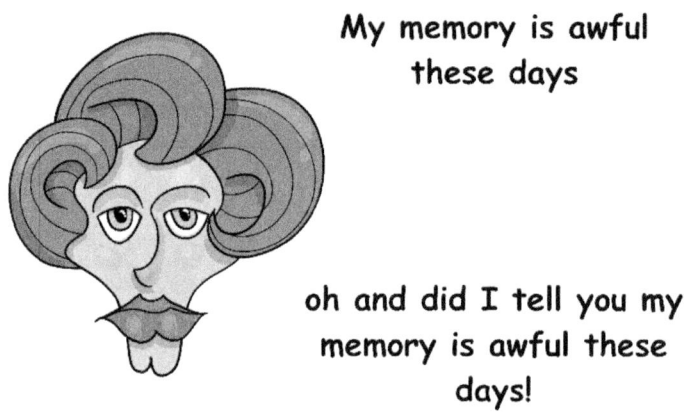

Figure 11: Photo

Several studies have shown that hormonal changes during menopause can impact brain structure and connectivity. Brain imaging studies found substantial differences in brain structure, connectivity, and energy metabolism across menopause stages (pre-menopause, peri-menopause, and post-menopause). These effects involved higher cognitive process-serving brain regions and were linked to cognitive performance. (Mosconi et al. 2021)

Other factors have been proposed as potential contributors to brain fog include:

Sleep Disturbance: Sleep is crucial for cognitive function and memory consolidation. Persistent disruptions can result in fatigue and reduced cognitive performance, contributing to brain fog.

Vascular Changes (meaning affecting blood vessels): Oestrogen also plays a role in maintaining vascular health, including blood flow regulation. Reduced oestrogen levels may affect blood flow in the brain, potentially impacting cognitive function.

Inflammation: Menopause is associated with an increase in inflammation around the body. Chronic inflammation can negatively impact brain function, leading to cognitive symptoms like brain fog.

Stress and Psycho-social Factors: The menopausal transition is often accompanied by increased stress and psychosocial challenges. Chronic stress can have detrimental effects on cognitive function and contribute to brain fog.

Ageing: As women age, other factors such as lifestyle habits (e.g. diet, physical activity), general health, and the ageing process itself can also influence cognitive function.

There is some evidence that social media attention deficits can contribute to menopausal brain fog. However, the exact relationship between the two is unknown. According to a survey conducted by Additude magazine, women with ADHD reported that brain fog or memory issues, as well as overwhelm, were the most impactful ADHD symptoms during menopause.

(https://www.additudemag.com/menopause-symptoms-adhd-survey/
https://www.additudemag.com/adhd-menopause-women-research/)

"I'd go from being sharp and focused, to just dull. Talking with other people was difficult because you can't focus, you can't understand what they're saying.

To stay focused, I had to jot down conversations, put little sticky notes everywhere, and just do tasks in smaller amounts so I wouldn't get overwhelmed and stressed which would add to the problem"

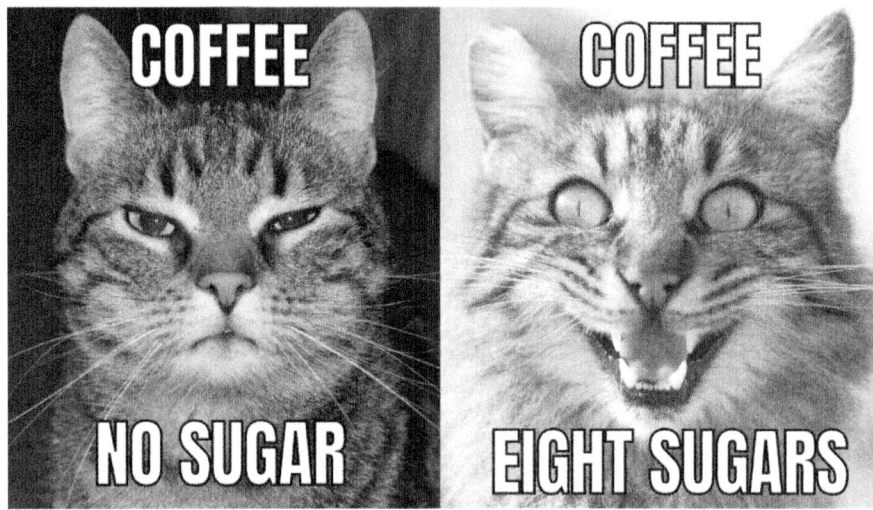

Figure 12: Photo

Role of Sugar in Brain Fog

Sugar gets a bad rap these days and while sugar is the primary energy source for cognitive functions, excessive sugar consumption has been linked to cognitive decline and brain fog.

The brain uses glucose, a type of sugar, as its primary energy source. Glucose is essential for the brain to function properly, and it is required for the production of neurotransmitters, which are the brain's chemical messengers. When there isn't enough glucose in the brain, neurotransmitters are not produced, and communication between neurons (brain nerves) breaks down. This can lead to cognitive decline and brain fog. (https://hms.harvard.edu/news-events/publications-archive/brain/sugar-brain)

Excessive sugar consumption can lead to metabolic disorders, such as insulin resistance and type 2 diabetes. Insulin is a hormone that helps to metabolise sugar in the body.

Insulin resistance is your body's cells resisting the normal effects of insulin. In other words, cells do not respond properly to insulin produced by your body or insulin administered as a medication. This causes the blood sugar levels to rise as it struggles to get out of the blood and into the tissues.

Eventually, insulin resistance may lead to Type 2 Diabetes. High blood sugar over time damages blood vessels in the brain that carry oxygen-rich blood. When the brain receives too little blood, brain cells shrink and can die. This is called brain atrophy and can cause problems with cognitive function and memory. (https://www.cdc.gov/diabetes/library/features/diabetes-and-your-brain.html)

Debunking myths

Myth 1: Menopausal Brain Fog Is Just a Normal Part of Ageing
You might have heard that brain fog during menopause is just another inevitable consequence of getting older. But here's the deal: it's not just about ageing. Hormonal changes during menopause play a significant role in those "senior moments" you might experience. Studies like the Women's Health Initiative Memory Study have revealed that it's the hormonal roller-coaster, not just the passage of time (Shumaker et al., 2003).

Myth 2: Brain Fog Only Affects Memory
While memory lapses are one part of the brain fog puzzle, this foggy state isn't limited to forgetting where you left your keys. Menopausal brain fog can also affect your ability to focus, make

decisions, and keep your thoughts in order. Again studies suggest that oestrogen is pulling the strings here in this cognitive arena (Greendale et al., 2009).

Myth 3: Nothing Can Be Done About Menopausal Brain Fog
There are strategies to help you manage and improve your brain fog. Please see the Action section of the book as we tackle how to help reduce Brain Fog. Hormone replacement therapy, when discussed with a healthcare provider, can be another piece of the puzzle.

Myth 4: All Women Will Experience Menopausal Brain Fog
Menopausal brain fog isn't a universal experience. The intensity and duration can vary from woman to woman. Factors like genetics, lifestyle, and overall health contribute to these differences. As the same question about brain fog to 10 different women, you will get 10 different answers, much like other menopausal symptoms.

Myth 5: Menopausal Brain Fog Is Irreversible
The good news is that menopausal brain fog isn't set in stone. Some cognitive aspects may bounce back post-menopause (Greendale et al., 2009). Engaging in brain-boosting activities, breathwork, maintaining a healthy lifestyle, and considering HRT can potentially help you regain your cognitive edge.

Myth 6: Cognitive Changes Are Always Negative
It's not all doom and gloom. Some women discover newfound creativity and better problem-solving skills during menopause. So, while the challenges are real, these changes can also be seen as an opportunity for personal growth and adaptation.

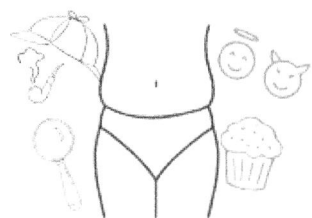

CHAPTER 8

THE MUFFIN
TOP MYSTERY:
Menopausal Weight Gain

I f there is one contentious area that is guaranteed to distress women, it's menopausal weight gain. It arrives like an uninvited guest that shows up at the worst possible time, bringing confusion, frustration and, causing a significant loss of confidence and self-shame.

As a woman's body undergoes this natural transition, it seems like the scale has a mind of its own, tipping the numbers in a direction that is never anticipated. Unfortunately weight gain is all too common a problem with over 50% of women complaining about it.

According to the SWAN study and the Healthy Women's study, women gain approximately 1.5kg per year during the perimenopause transition, resulting in an average weight gain of around about 10kg by the time menopause occurs.

When skin-folds and waist circumference were measured they indicated an increase in abdominal fat associated with menopause. However, HRT users didn't experience any changes in their mean weight, skin-fold thickness, or waist measurements. The study also suggests that body weight flattens out 2yrs after the final menstrual period.

(https://www.swanstudy.org/changes-in-body-composition-and-weight-during-the-menopause-transition/)

"I found it difficult to find actual information on how my body reacted to changes in hormone levels. I was told that my weight gain during the perimenopause was due to a change in my body's metabolism. No one told me that it is also due to me being less active and the way I drank, although I don't know how as I seem to be forever chasing around my husband and the kids. I thought I was active. I think I needed to have a good hard look at what I was doing and looking to eat better rather than just trying to stay slim all the time. We are so image-conscious all the time, sometimes it gets me down when I see other women managing their shape better than me"

Why why why!

Obesity and weight management in general is a complex area and is multifactorial in nature.

There are several factors contributing to the overall weight change and distribution of fat in the menopausal phases.

During perimenopause, the ovaries begin to produce less oestrogen. The latter helps regulate body weight by reducing insulin resistance and increasing energy expenditure. As levels decline, the body becomes less efficient at burning calories, which can lead to weight gain.

In addition to the increased total body fat and the different (negative) way fat is distributed around the body, loss of lean body mass (in other words muscle mass) and an expansion of fat tissue and re-distribution especially around the waist, increases the risk of metabolic diseases in women including type 2 diabetes and cardiovascular diseases.

Lack of oestrogen may interfere with the natural hunger signals your brain receives; it's been suggested that menopausal women experience greater hunger which encourages excessive food intake leading to weight gain.

In addition to oestrogen, other hormones such as the thyroid hormone, progesterone and testosterone also play a role in weight gain during menopause. An under or overactive thyroid will cause thyroid hormone fluctuations and so metabolic and calorie burning fluctuations. This may mean you putting on weight even though you are dieting and exercising. Progesterone helps regulate fluid balance in the body, and its fluctuations and decline can lead to water retention and bloating. Testosterone helps maintain muscle mass, and its decline can lead to a decrease in muscle mass and an increase in body fat. (Marsh et al. 2023, Chopra et al. 2019)

A woman's shape changes as her distribution of fat changes over the years, she moves from a more pear to apple shape. The same with men as their weight steadily increases from about 30 years of age and around the waist and abdomen. At the same time, their testosterone levels are steadily declining at approximately 1% per year which means muscle mass is dropping as well adding to the weight gain issue.

Both men and women lose muscle mass through the ageing process, this is known as **Sarcopenia**. However muscle mass influences how much energy your body uses in its normal day-to-day processes, in other words, its metabolism. The more muscle is lost, the less energy your body uses and so the greater the weight you are likely to keep.

There is a theory put forward in which it has been suggested that low-protein, highly processed foods lead to higher energy intake and therefore weight gain and obesity. It's been suggested there is an imbalance in micronutrient intake due to the body's powerful need for protein, which is being replaced by excessive consumption of fats and carbohydrates instead. (Zurlo et al. 1990, Grech et al. 2022)

Overall, one the best ways both men and women can help with their weight and satiety is to keep a high enough protein intake each meal, at least 20-25g of lean protein as well as keeping to a lower carbohydrate intake. This is alongside some form of resistance training to help preserve the existing muscle mass which is being lost through the ageing process.

Lifestyle factors such as alcohol intake and unhealthy eating behaviours, alongside medications and medical conditions such as thyroid disease, are also likely to contribute to weight gain in both men and women.

"I've been on HRT since April 2015 and began trying to lose weight in approximately September of the same year. It mostly fell off around about that time of year I remember, and I've spent ages trying to figure out how to maintain a normal stable weight since then, which I'm mostly doing okay now apart from the periodic yo-yoing. I'm not sure if the HRT made it easier or harder to lose weight, but it did make me feel less hungry for some reason. I just used an online programme that worked, but I reckon I could lose

another stone if I tried. I have also been encouraging my husband to lose some weight as well as his tummy seems to get bigger every time I see it!"

Role of HRT

HRT appears to have a conflicting role in weight management during the menopause. One analysis of over 100 trials with over 33,000 participants across 1.5 years found that HRT reduced abdominal obesity and increased lean body mass.

However, another analysis of 28 trials involving over 28,000 women suggested no evidence of an effect of HRT on body weight gain and not sufficient evidence on fat mass and distribution.

HRT has been shown to improve muscle strength. Despite preserving lean body mass at three years into the large WHI study, continuous long-term use of HRT at the six-year mark did not improve the loss of lean body mass with ageing. (Bea, J.W. et al. 2011, Kongnyuy et al. 2011,Salpeter et al. 2006)

Unfortunately, many women still report weight gain while taking Hormone Replacement Therapy. This may be due to other factors not involving HRT e.g., other medications and lifestyle issues, and should be investigated further.

As mentioned previously, oestrogen helps regulate body weight by reducing insulin resistance and increasing energy expenditure. However, as levels decline, the body becomes less efficient at burning calories, which can lead to weight gain.

HRT can also help increase energy levels, which can help relieve fatigue due to menopause, so women feel more energetic and can better manage their weight through diet and exercise. HRT can also help alleviate symptoms that interfere with weight loss, such as fatigue, sleep disturbances, and mood symptoms, and so indirectly allow women to make the choices necessary to shed unwanted pounds.

Managing Weight Gain

"Every time I looked in the mirror I knew I was getting heavier. I felt like a stuffed chicken in my dress. I knew I had to do something but I wasn't sure what exactly. My husband was trying a diet recommended by his personal trainer at his gym so I thought I try his. I could tell by the grin on his face that he'd got lucky, he knew I would do all the cooking for the both of us! I was 51 at the time and going through menopause. My doctor told me to come off the contraceptive pill so I did and I also started doing online Pilates and Zumba classes. There was no way I was going to join the gym in my state! I felt a lot better about myself when I started shifting the weight though. I knew I wasn't 20 and would never have that body again but I just didn't want to feel revolting anymore. My husband says I look a lot happier and more confident in myself now"

How should I start?

First of all, assess where you currently stand with your eating patterns and habits. If you are going to attempt weight loss, then government guidelines indicate a safe weight loss regime of 500Kcal per day, amounting to 3500Kcal per week. This is on top of some sort of exercise plan to help you to maintain the caloric deficit. Ask yourself the following:

Am I eating regularly or haphazardly?
What is my current diet like?

What is influencing my food choices and behaviours?
Do I eat on emotion?
What are my favourite healthy foods?
What unhealthy foods do I gravitate towards?
How big are my portions?
How often do I eat out?
How often do I cook at home?
Do I eat on the go?
Do I graze/snack unnecessarily?
Do I eat whilst trying to work or do other activities?
What are my biggest challenges when it comes to eating healthy?
How much water do I drink each day?
How much sugar do I consume each day?
How much protein do I consume each day?
How much fibre do I consume each day?
How much saturated fat do I consume each day?
How much sodium (salt) do I consume each day?
How much alcohol do I consume each week?
How much caffeine do I consume each day?
How much sleep do I get?
What are my favourite forms of exercise?
How often do I exercise?
What are my biggest challenges when it comes to exercising regularly?

The list can go on!

Asking yourself the hard questions with honest answers will either motivate you to take action or accept your current position. Understand here that as oestrogen levels decline so does muscle mass. As mentioned previously, there is also a redistribution of fat around the abdomen and upper body.

A key note here is that every woman is going through the changes, not just you. Please don't feel isolated here as if nature has singled you out in some sort of perverse weight management line up! The way you view your fluctuations in your weight going forward can have an impact on your quality of life because it is a very personal journey, and unique to you.

As a former Obesity Health Practitioner, I am aware that one of the main issues people have with their weight is that they insist on cutting out whole food groups at a time when they want to shed a few pounds, for example, the Ketogenic diet or the Soup diet.

Diet equals denial; what happens to people when they are denied anything, they crave it twice as badly. Unless you are super fastidious on your goal, It is simply easier to swap out the higher calorie density product in the food group with a lower one in the same food group.

For instance, instead of eating a whole bowl of french fries/chips with your meal, you could eat half of a bowl and replace the other half with more vegetables. By halving the amount of deep-fried potatoes you eat, you instantly reduce your calorie intake without depriving yourself of the chips. It is easier to do regular healthy swaps based on an 80/20 rule (where you are good 80% of the time) rather than following endless yo-yo dieting regimes.

Stay away from processed foods as they tend to lose most of their healthy nutrients through the manufacturing process. We are also duped by labelling and marketing. How often have you bought, say, an overpriced supermarket chicken salad because the pictures were nice, only to find very few pieces of chicken and a whole load of lettuce? This, accompanied by a high sugar, chemically manipulated dressing which is made to taste good by scientists but actually will leave you hungrier later on as your sugars crash and the hunger pangs arrive again.

Start with small changes and over time build up to bigger changes. A general rule I follow is that my plate should consist of 1/4 protein, 1/4 complex carbohydrates, 1/2 vegetables of all colours and textures, and a small amount of fat. There is no denial here and everything is homemade.

Protein and vegetables keep me fuller for longer reducing the need for snacking. Complex slow-release carbohydrates will mean a steady stream of fuel to the body and help maintain stable blood glucose, therefore insulin levels and hunger pangs. Fat keeps you satisfied; I finally finish off with fruit preferably low-carb berries which are also high in antioxidants.

Consume your food slowly (20 chews before swallowing) and know when you are **just full**, then just stop eating no matter what is left on the plate. By practising this technique you will soon understand how much food fills you up **just** at the point of fullness and no more. This prevents overeating, promotes discipline and just as importantly your brain registers how much you are eating. Your stomach has stretch receptors signalling to the brain when the stomach is full.

The habits around changing how you eat are meant to be implemented alongside exercising as well to help maintain your weight loss gains. This is paramount to keeping not only your weight in check, but also to help stave off other health challenges such as osteoporosis.

"Since I turned thirty five, I've noticed my energy has been steadily decreasing, and now that I'm in my mid-forties, I'm less sexually

active as well. I love my Chinese tea, but I've been consuming more tea—a different kind every day. Antioxidants found in tea are said to have health benefits. I'm eating less rice now that I can see a few extra pounds around my waist. To help tone my body, I work out every day"

While weight gain during menopause is common, there are steps women can take to manage it. Here are some tips:

• You've probably heard this a million times, **eat a healthy, balanced diet** that includes plenty of fruits, vegetables, whole grains, and lean protein. This is for good reason. Eating a rainbow of fruit and vegetables (that is all different colours and textures) will allow you to get a broad spectrum of beneficial chemicals and compounds found in nature.

This will also reduce your calorie intake by controlling portion size and prevent the use of cheap harmful food intake like low-quality oils, additives, etc. Making sure meals are homemade and not via takeaways will allow you to take firm control of the quality of ingredients that go into your mouth.

• **Keep up the protein levels** as it takes more energy to burn protein as well as helping to reduce muscle wastage due to the ageing process. At least 25g of protein should be eaten at every meal. This will keep you fuller for longer.

• **Stay Hydrated**: Water almost acts as a medicine in itself. Water is involved everywhere from the millions of chemical reactions going on in your body to making up tissue structure, reducing inflammation, improving cognition, and on and on.

Guidelines for daily intake will vary depending on the source, but aim for around 8 glasses of water a day, or as many as you can manage. You know when you are properly hydrated as your pee will be a natural straw colour and will lighten, the more you drink. A couple of bonuses are that your skin becomes more youthful looking and also your stomach will feel stretched so you're less likely to eat so much which will help you in weight management.

• **Limit** processed foods, sugary drinks, and alcohol. I think everybody knows this by now. Alcohol has a depressant action on the brain fuelling anxiety. Alcohol is also notoriously calorific in its content. A 175ml glass of wine is 2.3 units of alcohol and contains 159KCal; this is equivalent to 15.9 minutes running or eating half a cheeseburger.
(https://www.drinkaware.co.uk/tools/unit-and-calorie-calculator).

• **Engage** in regular physical activity, such as walking, swimming, or cycling. Start small and work your way up to any local health guidelines. Don't attempt to reach guidelines straight away as this may lead to overwhelm. Doing something is better than nothing.

• **Strength training** to maintain muscle mass. This is one of the best ways to keep a lid on your weight issues. The body has to use extra energy to help repair muscle tissue and prevent its breakdown all of which helps to burn fat. Resistance training helps to preserve the muscle tissue being lost as well as keeping you looking lean and toned.

Don't worry you are never going to look like a bodybuilder. Not only will that take years and years but you have to consume an obscene amount of calories to be that way. The goal here is to preserve muscle mass and build bone strength. The fabulous side effect will be weight loss, a stronger body, and a huge improvement in mood and bodily confidence.

• **Get enough sleep**. Lack of sleep has been linked to cravings, an increase in appetite for high-calorie foods, and a decrease in energy expenditure as well as affecting cortisol levels which influence your weight. We will look at sleep in the Action section of the book. (Papatriantafyllou et al. 2022).

• **Manage stress** through techniques such as meditation or yoga. whenever you get stressed your body releases cortisol to help combat stress. However, this hormone also stimulates fat and carbohydrate metabolism. This results in an energy surge in your body. While this process is necessary for survival, it also increases your appetite. High cortisol levels can also cause cravings for sweet, fatty, and salty foods; we also make bad food choices when we are stressed and on emotion.

• **Intermittent fasting**: Intermittent fasting is a pattern of eating that involves regular short-term fasts and consuming meals within a shorter period during the day, for example eating between 2 pm and 8 pm only.

This way of eating is effective in reducing body weight, ranging from 0.8% to 13.0% of baseline body weight. It is so simple to do, you are eating within only a set period of time. For example, I don't eat breakfast anymore, which means I ate my last meal at 8 pm the night before. My next meal will be at 2 pm lunchtime the next day. So I fast for 16hrs.

This is easy as most of the fasting is done while I am sleeping and I use black coffee in the mornings to get me through til lunchtime. If you are overweight then this is a great strategy to use on a short-term basis. Fasting is also a great way to improve Insulin sensitivity, reducing your risk of Type 2 Diabetes, cardiovascular diseases, etc. (Welton et al. 2020).

• **Behaviour therapy**, including self-monitoring, goal setting, and problem-solving, can also help promote healthy eating habits and weight management. Check out the **www.sisstas.com** website for weight loss challenges.

• **Calorie tracking** and self-monitoring: Self-monitoring is a critical factor in successfully losing weight. People can use a paper diary, mobile app, or dedicated website to record items of food that they consume each day. They can also measure their progress by recording their weight every week or simply by the clothes they wear. Self-monitoring can help increase awareness of eating habits, promote accountability, and facilitate behaviour change. (Burke, 2011).

• **Reducing carbohydrate intake**: Reducing carbohydrate intake can be an effective strategy for weight loss and weight maintenance. Low-carbohydrate diets are effective in promoting weight loss and improving metabolic health markers such as blood pressure, blood glucose, and cholesterol levels. Note that the Ketogenic diet is a very low carbohydrate diet, less than 5% carbohydrate with a predominantly high fat intake. Although this diet is also an effective way of shedding pounds, it does come with issues such as gall bladder problems, so please seek medical advice before starting any Keto diet.

It is important to note that not all carbohydrates are created equal, and a diet rich in whole grains, fruits, and vegetables can provide essential nutrients and promote overall health rather than a diet of pizzas, burgers, and chips. These tend to be higher in processed cheap carbohydrates which are damaging to the body as well as weight-promoting.

"I had heard soya may be beneficial for some women, so I changed my diet primarily to only drink calcium-fortified soy milk in my tea, coffee, and cereal. I believe this has helped lessen the severity of my daytime sweats"

Obesity and weight gain are complicated areas. I could write a whole book just on this topic alone. If you are concerned about your weight and how to eat moving forward, I would suggest you speak to either a nutritionist or a dietitian. This will be a great investment not only in your weight but in your overall health.

There are many strategies women can use to help maintain or lower their weight, so weight gain during menopause doesn't have to be inevitable. Don't wait for a knight in shining armour that will never come to rescue you, find it in yourself to incorporate exercise and healthy choices in your lifestyle.

Eating for Menopause

Your diet can either promote/cause disease, think diabetes, or favour/prevent disease for example, scurvy due to a lack of vitamin C frequently experienced by sailors during the "Age of Exploration", (between the 1500s and 1800s). Whilst the vast majority of women hone in on their weight as their main problem, their real focus should be on preventing the onset of diseases as they age. The prevalence of conditions such as osteoporosis, cardiovascular disease, and metabolic diseases such as diabetes increase as women move through all phases of the menopause cycle.

It is now globally accepted that two of the best patterns of eating to follow are The Mediterranean and the Asiatic diets. This is because they have been widely researched and accepted as having excellent nutritive and health profiles. In the menopausal age group, we should be looking at foods as functional medicines rather than just fuel. Bioactive compounds which are present in many plant-based foods can positively help the body's physiology and contribute towards disease prevention. Here are a few to be aware of:

Polyphenols: Found in plants, they provide their pigmentation, colour and an antioxidant role. Diets high in polyphenols, particularly flavonoids from foods like soy and tea, can improve health by reducing the physiological effects and symptoms of menopause. Japanese women are a testament to that. They have fewer symptoms and it's generally attributed to their diet. Other flavonoid-containing diets and supplements, like isoflavones (phytoestrogens), mimic the effects of oestrogen. Their chemical structure is similar and they may be of particular benefit when consumed regularly. Consuming polyphenols may help delay the ageing process during the menopausal phase.

Example foods include blueberries, plums, cherries, apples, strawberries, black currants, black olives, dark chocolate, black tea, coffee, hazelnuts, and pecans.
(https://www.uclahealth.org/news/polyphenols)

Soy protein and isoflavone consumption may help postmenopausal women reduce bone loss, reduce calcium in their urine, and increase their bone mineral density. These include soy milk and butter, tofu, edamame beans, soybeans, tempeh, miso, ramen, natto. The potential benefit of adding probiotics containing lactobacillus and bifidobacterium to soy milk is that they may increase the absorption and bioavailability of calcium.

Antioxidants like beta-carotene, as well as vitamins C and E, protect from the damaging effects of oxidative stress which is a chemical reaction promoting ageing. Magnesium improves energy metabolism, transport across cells, skeletal muscle function, and of course sleep. Studies have also found high intakes of fruit and vegetables rich in a variety of carotenoids might provide benefits to bone health in postmenopausal Japanese females. (C.J.H. Martin et al. 2013)

"I completely changed my diet and started working out every day. I also went plant-based, making sure they were whole foods, adding legumes as a main source of protein, eating more vegetables, and, whenever possible, avoiding processed foods and sugar. I wasn't a goody two shoes all the time but I made my peace with that and I felt great"

The Mediterranean diet focuses on a diet that is rich in foods with anti-inflammatory and antioxidant properties, such as extra-virgin olive oil, vegetables, fruits, legumes, nuts, and whole-grain cereals, which can contribute to weight control. It is lower in meat, moderate in fish, and lowest in consumed sweetened beverages; all of which promote heart health and also reduce insulin resistance.

I would also add that this style of eating may be easier to follow because ingredients may be more readily available than Asian ones but are not lacking in variety or flavour. This type of diet benefits cardiac health, bone health, and cognition due to its omega-fatty acid content and weight management.

Phytoestrogens mimic the effects of natural oestrogen in the body because of their chemical structure but are weaker in nature. Common foods include flaxseed, chia seeds, tofu and soy, sprouts, garlic, peaches, wheat bran, chickpeas, and almonds. Studies have shown a short-term but large dose of dietary phytoestrogen supplementation can significantly relieve the severity of hot flushes and vaginal dryness in menopausal women as well as benefit osteoporosis. A contemporary strategy for preventing postmenopausal osteoporosis is based on diet, exercise, and exposure to sunlight. (Brzezinski et al. 1997).

Potassium, which is found in fruits and legumes, has an alkalising effect that can stop the elimination of calcium from bones through the urine. Vitamin K, which enhances bone metabolism, is especially found in green leafy vegetables. A good combination is vitamin D, calcium, and vitamin K if there is a deficiency. However, check with your pharmacist in case there are any issues with medications.

Turmeric has been used for centuries as a dietary spice, as well as a traditional Ayurvedic remedy to treat numerous common ailments in India. It has also been used in China and Arabia. It is Polyphenol derived from the Curcuma Longa (from the ginger family) plant, the active ingredient being Curcumin. Among the health benefits of this well-known spice, it has been suggested that menopausal women may benefit from increased libido, decreased arthritic pain, better cognition, and fewer hot flushes. As it is poorly absorbed, taking Curcumin with pepper will improve its absorption.

But the advantages that Indians experience stem from their regular consumption of Curcumin, not from using it as a one-time remedy.

This spice can be added to curries, soups, stews, smoothies, milk, teas, and as a marinade.

Another powerful antioxidant is **Quercetin.** It is found in the following foods: grapes, berries, cherries, apples, citrus fruits, onions, buckwheat, kale, tomatoes, red wine, and black tea. It appears to have many beneficial properties including antidiabetic, anti-inflammatory, antioxidant, antimicrobial, anti-Alzheimer's, anti-arthritic, cardiovascular, and wound-healing effects. (Salehi et al. 2020)

The last compound I will highlight is **Chlorogenic acid.** This is another polyphenol chemical that is a common ingredient in plant-based foods and has gained a lot of attention because of its antiviral, antibacterial, anti-inflammatory, and antioxidant properties. It contributes to better insulin resistance, controlling the metabolism of fats and carbohydrates, and lowering the risk of type 2 diabetes and cardiovascular illnesses.

It can be found in tea, coffee, and certain foods and herbs, like apples, carrots, eggplants, betel, honeysuckle, artichokes potatoes, pears, plums, and grapes (Santana-Gálvez et al. 2017)

Of course, there are going to be many more compounds on the list but this is not a science lecture. I wanted to highlight perhaps the most researched and well-known. These compounds are also studied for their potential as therapeutic molecules in designing future medicines for some of the conditions mentioned above.

A great resource is provided by the British Dietetic Association for Menopausal Eating.
https://www.bda.uk.com/resource/menopause-diet.html

The British and Irish Hypertension Charity with their healthy eating sheet can be found under their miscellaneous section, and typing in healthy eating.
https://bihsoc.org/resources/miscellaneous/

As a minimum, I used to suggest that women have an adequate amount of vitamin D, calcium, vitamin K, omega fatty acids both 3 and 6 in balance, and B vitamins especially 6 (for periods) and 12 (for cognition), so a B complex (also for energy) would cover them all. Minerals such as zinc (immunity) magnesium (sleep) selenium (hair and nails, but toxic in large doses), and chromium (blood sugar stability). It becomes difficult to recommend dosages as this will vary from health jurisdictions and health organisations.

Have a chat with your pharmacist or health food store assistant who should give you more guidance on supplementation.

A healthy balanced diet will cover all of these vitamins and minerals.

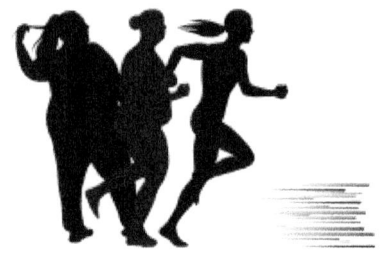

CHAPTER 9

STAY FIT, STAY FLAB-U-LESS:
Menopausal Physical Activity

"Take care of your body. It's the only place you have to live."

- Jim Rohn

The importance of physical activity cannot be underestimated. We are designed by nature to be active and not sedentary creatures.

Physical activity and weight management go hand in hand. Exercise is known for its ability to keep the human body lean, promote a sense of well-being, and lift mood.

There are numerous benefits of exercise from stress reduction to strengthening bones for both men and women and clearing of toxins and dead cells through increased circulation in the body.

In both men and women after the age of 40, muscle mass is being lost through the ageing process (Sarcopenia), resistance training with an adequate amount of protein intake improves metabolism and can help build up lost muscle whilst at the same time firing up fat burning.

There is no conclusive evidence derived from randomised trials on whether exercise is an effective treatment for reducing hot flushes and night sweats in menopausal women. Evidence can be conflicting depending on the studies that are examined. However, sedentary women are more likely to experience menopause symptoms than active women. (Romani et al. 2009)

The Benefits of Physical Activity During Menopause

There are so many benefits for menopausal women when they participate in regular physical activity. Here are some of the most important ones:

Improved Mood and Mental Health: Menopause can be a challenging time for many women, and it can lead to feelings of anxiety, depression, and irritability. Exercise has been shown to improve mood and reduce symptoms of anxiety and depression. (Sternfeld et al.2011)

Improved Sleep: Sleep disturbances are a common symptom of menopause, and they can have a significant impact on a woman's quality of life. Exercise improves sleep quality and reduces the frequency of sleep disturbances. (Dąbrowska et al. 2016).

Reduced Risk of Chronic Diseases: Menopause is associated with an increased risk of chronic diseases such as heart disease, osteoporosis, and type 2 diabetes. Regular physical activity can help reduce the risk of these diseases and improve overall health.(Mishra et al. 2011).

Weight Management: Menopause can lead to weight gain, particularly around the midsection. Regular physical activity can help manage weight and reduce the risk of obesity. I think most people know this by now.

Improved Bone Health: Menopause is associated with a decline in bone density, which can lead to osteoporosis and an increased risk of fractures. Weight-bearing exercises such as walking, jogging, and strength training can help improve bone density and reduce the risk of fractures. (Benedetti et al. 2010).

Current UK NHS guidelines state adults should engage in at least 150 minutes of moderate-intensity, or 75 minutes of vigorous-intensity exercise per week. This is especially true for women experiencing menopausal symptoms. Your weekly exercises can be divided into small sessions, a combination of both, or all at once. Even if you can't meet the guidelines, any amount of physical activity is better than none. Just small increases in activity can have significant health benefits.

Many different types of physical activity can be beneficial during menopause. Here are some examples:

Aerobic Exercise: Aerobic exercise, also known as cardio, is any activity that increases your heart rate and breathing rate. Examples include brisk walking, jogging, cycling, swimming, and dancing. Aerobic exercise can improve cardiovascular health, reduce the risk of chronic diseases, and improve mood and mental health.

Strength Training: Strength training, also known as resistance training, involves using weights or resistance bands to build muscle strength and endurance. Strength training can improve bone density, reduce the risk of falls, and improve overall physical function.

Yoga and Pilates: Yoga and Pilates are low-impact exercises that focus on flexibility, balance, and core strength. These exercises can improve flexibility, reduce stress, and improve overall physicality.

Pelvic Floor Exercises: Pelvic floor exercises, also known as Kegels, involve contracting and relaxing the muscles of the pelvic floor. These exercises can improve bladder control and reduce the risk of urinary incontinence. (https://www.stelizabeth.com/healthyheadlines/why-exercise-is-good-medicine-for-menopause-symptoms/)

Note the online programme of this book has demonstrations of Yoga, Breathing, and Kegel Exercises specific to menopause, performed by suitably qualified practitioners.

If you're new to exercise or haven't exercised in a while, it's important to start slowly and gradually increase the intensity and duration of your workouts. Here are some tips to help you get started:

Important! Before starting any exercise programme, it's important to consult with your doctor first, This is particularly important in menopausal women as they are at risk of low bone density and therefore fractures.

Start Slowly: Begin with low-intensity activities such as walking or gentle yoga and gradually increase the intensity and duration of your workouts.

Find Activities You Enjoy: Choose activities that you enjoy and that fit into your lifestyle. This will make it easier to stick with your exercise programme.

Mix It Up: Incorporate a variety of activities into your exercise programme to keep it interesting and challenging.

Set Realistic Goals: Set realistic goals for yourself and vitally, celebrate your progress along the way.

"I was so overweight I was unable to sleep at night because I kept having these thoughts of not making it to 60. My husband was supportive but I could tell he wasn't attracted to me anymore. I knew I had to do something. At first, when I joined the gym I felt ugly and ashamed, I remember not being able to do any push-ups or any type of crawling exercise as I would get out of breath. I got talking to the female personal trainer whom I started working with each week, she got me an eating plan, and eventually, after about 5 months of persevering, I lost over 80 pounds, which to this day I still can't believe. Not only did I feel great but my love life improved as well, I had a much smaller tyre around the middle and I felt a lot more confident and just more alive. I now work out with a small group of friends and go on evening runs with a local club. It's great, I finally feel good about myself"

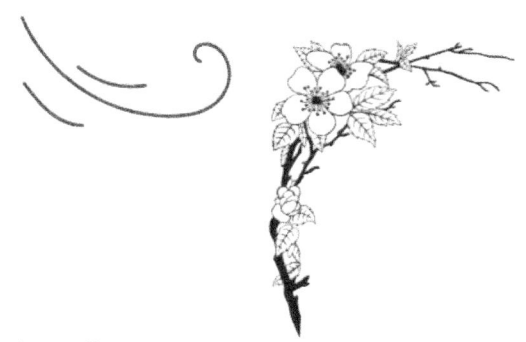

CHAPTER 10

WEATHERING HER MENOPAUSE TSUNAMI:
How Men Can Help

Manning Up!

Men can play a critical role in supporting women through their menopausal symptoms by understanding what menopause is, and how it can affect women's physical, emotional, and psychological health. Men, this is for you. Here are some ways you can be more supportive towards your partner's menopausal symptoms:

1. Educate yourself about menopause

It's easy to be blase about it and roll your eyes every time she complains, but this is a serious and major turning point in a woman's life and it's not going away!

A detailed overview is the first part of this book, but a very brief summary could be as follows:

- Menopause is a natural process that marks the end of a woman's reproductive years. It typically occurs between the ages of 45 and 55, but can happen earlier or later. It can lead to a range of debilitating symptoms, including hot flushes, night sweats, mood swings(anxiety and depression), sleep and weight changes, joint aches and pains, skin issues, vaginal dryness and osteoporosis
- It is caused by a dramatic shift in hormones, the main loss being Oestrogen and an overall imbalance of hormones in general, which leads to the issues mentioned above. It can be a natural menopause as nature intended or suddenly as a consequence of surgery, chemicals e.g., medications including chemotherapy. It can last for many years anywhere from approximately 4-10.
- There are many other glands in the body that are involved such as the Thyroid, which means symptoms widely vary from person to person. Menopausal symptoms can be managed with medications such as HRT or non-drug based complimentary therapies and supplements as well as exercise and diet.

What the menopause is not is time of the month! it's actually worse as it is ongoing with seemingly no signs of stopping.

A menopausal sufferer cannot just snap out of her mood swing or over exaggerate her poor sleep; the menopause represents a loss of control both physically and emotionally, and the best way forward is to have an understanding of what is happening to her and have some sort of plan that you can map out together moving forward.

Remember this is a small investment for you that is likely to pay off in the long run.

We have already mentioned some of the typical symptoms which would include:

- hot flushes, heart racing palpitations and night sweats
- fatigue, insomnia and sleep disturbances
- poor concentration and brain fog
- dry eyes, aching joints and headaches
- hair loss and skin irritation e.g. itchiness and dryness
- urinary issues, loss of libido, vaginal issues e.g. dryness or itchiness
- changes to periods such as irregular, heavy or painful

There may also be associated psychological symptoms including:

- anxiety depression and panic attacks
- mood swings and irritability
- reduced or loss of confidence of confidence

Many women do not always recognise that they are experiencing symptoms because they may still be having regular periods when they first start to experience them.

2. Give her "me" time

Women continue to juggle both family and work pressures, which leaves little time for their own priorities.

In today's busy environment, where everyone is scrambling to find time it can be challenging to carve it out.

Giving her "me" time means giving her space and time for self care and mental health.

If for example she needs time to do yoga in the morning, you can provide that space for her and take over the activities she would normally do.

This is hugely important as it has a dramatic impact on how her interpretation of the menopause change is going to be. If she has a more positive outlook then she is likely to have a far better experience of it, and so making your life easier in the long run.

Now let's face it you are not going to be able to help her every single minute of the day and on every whim. Just remember your only providing support, you cannot take the menopause away from her, but the way you provide support will have a significant impact in her life.

3. Acknowledge the situation

As frustrating as her symptoms maybe, acknowledge it and discuss in an empathetic manner, how you can help. Don't roll your eyes and try and bite your tongue where you can; this is not easy for her either as there is a hormonal storm going on inside her right now.

Use open ended questions to find out what the issues are and ask her what she expect you to do about it.

Questions start that start with "what" "how or "why" will encourage a fuller answer, rather than the "yes" or "no" response from a closed-ended question.

e.g.,

How are you feeling today?

What can I do to make this better?

Why do you think you got stressed today?

Consider what is being stated as you listen. Don't try to fix the issue or downplay their response or feelings, just listen.

4. Help with household chores

Women going through menopause may experience fatigue and other physical symptoms, making it challenging for them to do everyday tasks. You can help by offering to take on more household chores, such as cleaning, cooking, or grocery shopping. This is an opportunity to show your partner you are there for them.

5. Encourage physical activity

Exercise can help with some of the menopausal symptoms, such as mood swings, and weight gain. Men can encourage women to exercise regularly and offer to join them on walks or other physical activities. This is important for both men and women. As we age, our muscle mass and strength tend to decline, which can lead to decreased mobility and independence.

Engaging in regular physical activity can help maintain muscle mass and strength, as well as flexibility and range of motion, which can improve overall physical function and reduce the risk of falls and injuries.

Exercise has numerous other benefits such as improving mental health, reducing risk of chronic diseases, improving cognition and maintaining a healthy weight.

According to research, couples who engage in novel and interesting activities together express greater satisfaction and love for their partners. (Aron et al. 2000)

It's also likely that exercise increases physical attraction towards each other as well as strengthen your bonds.

Suggest an activity that you could do together, it doesn't have to be strenuous; anything from walking or jogging. It can be anything you like as long as it involves physical movement that you are doing together and for a specified length of time for example, an hour.

6. Listen and communicate effectively

Here are some general tips that may be helpful if you need them:

Practise active listening: This means giving her your full attention, showing that you are listening and understanding what she is saying. You can do this by maintaining eye contact, nodding your head, and asking follow-up questions.

Avoid interrupting: Interrupting can be seen as disrespectful and can hinder effective communication. Wait for her to finish speaking before you respond.

Validate her feelings: Women often want to feel heard and understood. You can do this by acknowledging her emotions and validating her feelings. For example, "I can understand why you feel that way" or "That must have been difficult for you."

Avoid being defensive or dismissive: It's important to approach conversations with an open mind and a willingness to learn. If she says something you don't agree with, ask for clarification or try to see things from her perspective.

When expressing your own thoughts or feelings, try to use "I" statements instead of "you" statements. For example, instead of saying "You're wrong," say "I see things differently."

Here are some additional resources that may be helpful:

"The Art of Listening" by Michael P. Nichols: This book provides practical tips and techniques for effective communication and active listening.

"Men Are from Mars, Women Are from Venus" by John Gray: This book explores the differences in communication styles between men and women and offers advice for improving communication in relationships.

It took me a while to remember that communication is a skill that takes practise and effort to develop. By being attentive, empathetic, and open-minded, you can improve your ability to communicate effectively.

It's essential to create an open and supportive environment where women feel comfortable discussing their menopause symptoms.

Non verbal cues such as showing affection by offering hugs, holding hands, can go a long way in making women feel better during this challenging time.

7. Discussing other options

Take the time to look at and explore other options with her. There are a wide range of complimentary medicines, holistic practises such as reflexology, herbs and supplements that maybe of benefit.

Perhaps you could accompany her in discussions with the medical or alternative health practitioner. Make her feel your support just by being present and open to suggestions.

Please be aware that the menopause will accelerate conditions like osteoporosis (which happens in men too) so it's important to think about the long term challenges you may face by not doing something early.

Perhaps come up with a commitment contract that you can put on the fridge that reminds you of your obligations towards her.

Here is an example I jokingly wrote out for myself to use:

NON-BINDING NON-LEGAL AGREEMENT FOR HUSBAND TO HELP WITH WIFE'S MENOPAUSAL SYMPTOMS

This agreement made on [date], between [Husband's Name], referred to as the "Husband," and [Wife's Name], referred to as the "Wife."

The parties agree as follows:

1. The Husband recognises that the Wife is experiencing menopausal symptoms, which may include but are not limited to hot flushes, night sweats, mood swings, and sleep disturbances.

2. The Husband commits to helping the Wife manage these symptoms to the best of his ability, with the understanding that he is not a medical professional and cannot provide medical advice or treatment.

3. The Husband will make an effort to be understanding and patient with the Wife during this time, recognising that menopause can be a challenging and sometimes frustrating experience.

4. The Husband will assist the Wife with tasks or activities that may be difficult for her due to her symptoms, such as cooking, cleaning, or running errands. The Husband will also engage in activities together with the wife that may help her reduce or alleviate her symptoms such as exercise or weight control.

5. The Wife acknowledges that her symptoms may vary in intensity and frequency, and that the Husband's ability to help may also vary depending on his own schedule and commitments and personal abilities. The Wife will also acknowledge that the

Husband will commit to the best of his abilities and will look for progress in his actions rather than perfection.

6. This agreement is non-binding, has no value in any court of law in any state or country and not is intended to create any legal obligations or liabilities for either party.

7. Either party may terminate this agreement at any time by providing either verbal or written notice to the other party.

8. This agreement represents the understanding and agreement of the parties and supersedes all prior negotiations, understandings, and agreements between the parties.

Signed on this [date],

....

Husband's Name...............

Wife's Name..................

This module was written to help create an understanding of where a husband or partner could play a greater role in supporting and alleviating some of the symptoms of the menopause, their partners maybe facing.

Don't expect to be perfect at this, I'm certainly not, but I do recognise where I maybe of help.

Hopefully you have found the information useful and in someway contributes to a more harmonious household.

Good Luck!

Male Menopause: Myth or Reality?

Men are notorious for keeping things to themselves especially in matters of health. It's likely you may not have heard of the male menopause and limited to stories if any on erectile dysfunction.

The existence of the Male Menopause or Andropause is still a matter of debate in the medical community. Unlike menopause in women, which is a well-defined period marked by a sudden drop in hormone levels, the decline in testosterone levels in men is gradual and occurs over a longer period.

Some doctors refer to this condition as androgen decline in the ageing male or low testosterone. A late-onset hypogonadism is a testosterone deficiency that develops later in life.

However, many men experience symptoms associated with male menopause, and it is important to understand how to manage them.

Symptoms of Male Menopause

The symptoms of male menopause can vary from person to person, but some of the most common ones include:

Fatigue
Low sex drive
Erectile dysfunction
Depression or sadness
Decreased motivation
Lowered self-confidence
Difficulty concentrating
Insomnia or difficulty sleeping
Increased body fat
Loss of Muscle Mass
Man boobs (gynaecomastia)
Large belly

Unlike women who experience a more rapid change in hormone status during the menopause, testosterone decline is steady at about 1% per year between the ages of 30 and 40, and because the change is gradual this is unlikely to cause any problems in and of itself.

Total testosterone is measured in nanomoles per litre (nmol/l) in the UK, but nanograms per deciliter (ng/dL) is the preferred unit in the US. So what is the 'normal' range in a man of 70 won't be the same as that for a man at the age of 40, yet the standard ranges usually do not take account of this factor.

It also seems that symptoms maybe expressed at different levels of testosterone, for example loss of energy maybe at a higher level of testosterone than say depression.

(centreformenshealth.co.uk)

The decline in testosterone levels during male menopause can have a significant impact on mental health. Some of the most common mental health symptoms associated with male menopause include:

Low self-esteem
Relationship problems
Depression

Unfortunately, the fact that testosterone and hormonal balance are important to a healthy mental state means that thousands of men experience negative mental health effects at the hands of the male menopause each year. With the condition often going undiagnosed, this is a huge problem. If you are experiencing or think that you are experiencing the male menopause after reading this then a medical practitioner like an endocrinologist really needs to be involved for an accurate diagnosis. Again don't suffer in silence, take action for a better quality of life.

Ideally a complete physical examination plus blood tests as well as an examination of the source of symptoms will provide an accurate picture of what is going on.

If a specialist confirms a male menopause diagnosis, you may be prescribed testosterone replacement therapy in order to correct the hormone deficiency. The testosterone replacement treatment normally comes as an injection or as a gel here in the UK. This should alleviate the symptoms.

However, it is important to note that replacement therapy is not suitable for everyone, and it can have side effects such as acne, breast enlargement, and an increased risk of blood clots.

Lifestyle changes that men can make to manage the symptoms of male menopause include:

Regular exercise: This one is very important. Exercise can help improve mood, increase energy levels, and reduce body fat. Testosterone is also needed to maintain muscle mass due to age related loss of muscle also known as sarcopenia. Exercise, especially resistance training, boosts growth hormone levels and testosterone levels which helps preserve skeletal mass.

Healthy eating: A balanced diet that is low in sugar, salt, and unhealthy fats can help manage weight and reduce the risk of obesity.

Stress management: Stress can exacerbate the symptoms of male menopause. Techniques such as meditation, yoga, and deep breathing can help reduce stress levels.

Good sleep hygiene: Getting enough sleep is important for overall health and well-being. Men can improve their sleep hygiene by establishing a regular sleep schedule, avoiding caffeine and alcohol before bedtime, and creating a relaxing sleep environment.

While there is no scientific data to support the belief that food can boost testosterone levels, there are many foods that are rich in certain micronutrients that are believed to be beneficial for trying to boost testosterone levels. Here are some of the most commonly cited testosterone-boosting foods:

Eggs
Avocados
Bananas
Oysters and shellfish
Pomegranates, cherries, berries
Almonds
Ginger
Fatty fish such as tuna, mackerel, salmon, sardines, tilapia, and trout
Leafy greens such as spinach and kale
Garlic
Meat
Fruit
Cocoa
Berries
Egg yolks
White button mushrooms
Red meat

It's important to note that overall lifestyle is more important for testosterone levels than singular foods. (Bailey 2023, Leonard 2023).

"Dear Reader, If you're enjoying this book, I'd be immensely grateful if you could spare a moment (literally 5 seconds) to share your thoughts with others on Amazon. Positive reviews from wonderful customers like you can make a huge difference and help empower other readers in their menopausal journey. Thank you deeply for your kind words, time and support!"

Please see page 265 for details

CONCLUSION

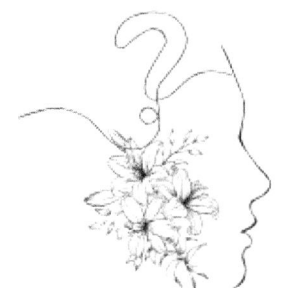

As I wrap up sharing my thoughts about the menopause, I feel like I'm closing a chapter on a journey full of ups and downs and surprises. Especially from the conversations I have had with regular women with everyday challenges.

In my humble opinion – menopause isn't a one-size-fits-all thing. It's more like a crazy, unique journey that every woman goes through in her own way. I've learned that it's not about fighting against the changes but figuring out how to work with your body's own rhythm.

We've talked about the wild ride of hormones, and the not-so-friendly changes in your body. But just remember, these aren't enemies; they're just your body's way of throwing you a curveball. And maybe, it's time to start seeing them as signals to slow down, listen, and show yourself a little kindness.

Self-care isn't a luxury – it's a must. Whether it's choosing good nutrition, getting moving, or taking a moment to breathe, it's about saying, "Hey, I'm worth it." And let me tell you, surrounding yourself with a group of friends, family, or experts who understand it makes a world of difference. Laughter, shared experiences, and sometimes a good cry – they all make the journey a bit easier.

Menopause isn't about fading away; it's about growing into a version of yourself you've never met before. It's about knowing more, loving yourself better, and stepping into whatever comes next with arms wide open.

We are now moving onto the Action section of this book.

"So many women I've talked to see menopause as an ending. But I've discovered this is your moment to reinvent yourself after years of focusing on the needs of everyone else. It's your opportunity to get clear about what matters to you and then to pursue that with all of your energy, time and talent." — Oprah Winfrey

TAKING ACTION

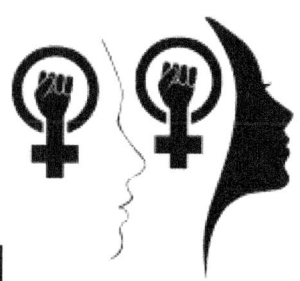

"The path to success is to take massive, determined actions"

- Tony Robbins

The first part of this book focused on knowledge and awareness of what was happening during menopause to your body and the associated symptoms that came with it.

We are now progressing into the Action Section of the book. Our focus now is to manage the below symptoms by reducing their intensity and frequency and in general improving the quality of your life:

Hot Flushes Night Sweats and Improved Sleep
Joint Pain
Brain Fog
Fatigue
Genito-Urinary Issues

This is the most important part of the book and what you have paid your hard earned money for. This is about taking massive action to manage and relieve your symptoms.

Self help however takes a certain mindset. It's about moving forward with only you being accountable for your actions. It is no good buying a self-help book only to find the good intentions you had only lasted a week, and progress is not as fast as you think it was going to be, or worse, just buying a book and leaving it to gather dust. There is no medication here to provide immediate relief, but also, there is no risk and awful side effects that medications may present as well. Anything that involves the body takes time, focus, and practise. You are the most important person here and self-care is required but it should not be seen as selfish care.

This book and the **online programme at www.sisstas.com** are designed to treat a particular symptom over a 4-6 week period. It's a "boot camp" style course to speed up the relief of your symptoms by applying maximum effort on the part of the participant. We all have that little voice in our heads that whispers, "You can't do it." These self-limiting beliefs can hold us back from reaching our full potential. But here's the thing – they're just thoughts, not facts. By recognising and challenging these negative beliefs, you can break free from their grip and open yourself up to a world of possibilities. Unfortunately, menopause has many negative connotations in the West, but how you approach it moving forward can have a significant impact on your quality of life.

Everything you are about to try is evidence-based and does work with continuous practise. Results will always fluctuate between individuals, but perseverance is the name of the game here. As part of the hypnosis sessions we have with the online programme, visualising your success can help you achieve it.

It might sound a little woo-woo, but many successful athletes, entrepreneurs, and artists swear by the power of hypnosis and visualisation. By repeating to yourself and imagining in your mind reaching your goals and experiencing the feelings of success, you can programme your mind to work towards making those visions a reality. As a certified hypnotherapist, I know this stuff works if you allow it to.

I would encourage you to adopt a growth mindset here. This is where you believe that your abilities aren't innate but can be improved through effort, learning, and persistence. When you adopt a growth mindset, you see challenges as opportunities to learn and grow, rather than as roadblocks to your success. Studies in psychology have indicated that individuals with a growth mindset are more likely to embrace challenges, persist in the face of setbacks, and ultimately achieve higher levels of success.

Sure you are going to have your bad days, your children are going to annoy you, you're running late and don't have time to do the yoga in the morning, you just can't be bothered to go lower carb today, and so on. Life is full of ups and downs, and setbacks are bound to happen along the way. But it's not the setbacks that define us – it's how we bounce back from them. Developing resilience is key to overcoming obstacles and staying on track towards your goals. Resilient individuals can adapt to change, bounce back from failure, and keep moving forward, no matter what life throws their way.

Try and keep to an 80/20 principle, where you succeed in committing 80% of the time but a 20% failure is acceptable and you're not beating yourself up about it.

And finally, in this very short mindset blurb, try and surround yourself with positive individuals who either understand what is going on with menopause, or at least those who are going through the change with you.

By surrounding yourself with individuals who understand your issues and share your values and aspirations, you can create a positive feedback loop of motivation and inspiration, moving you toward your goals with unwavering support and encouragement. There are plenty of support groups around this area of health, please think about joining one if you haven't already done so.

Let us begin:

The Action section is going to be broken down into 3 main areas:

- **The Tools**
- **The Roadmap**
- **Implementation and Progress Monitoring**

TOOLS

Let's examine these first. Throughout the programme we are going to rely on the following:

- Breathwork (Paced Breathing and Pranayama) - for fatigue, stress reduction, pain relief, hot flushes, improved sleep and brain fog
- Yoga – for joint pain, stress reduction, improved sleep, fatigue
- Focused Mindfulness – for brain fog and concentration, pain relief
- Pelvic Floor Exercises (Kegel Exercises) - for genito-urinary issues
- Cognitive Behavioural Therapy (CBT) - for hot flushes, pain relief, anxiety
- Changes in Eating Patterns

Important! **Remember to check you are medically fit to use the tools mentioned.**

Over time, try and use as many tools as possible because they will have indirect and overlapping benefits. For example, if you are treating joint pain, then yoga will be of great benefit but also, using the breathwork will reduce your stress which in turn reduces muscle tightening and decreasing pain sensitivity. This is a matter of experimentation to see what works for you.

Please remember to introduce the tools slowly over the weeks. There is no race here, I want you to be able to incorporate them into your busy lifestyles. Don't try them all at once, bring them in over a week or so.

How you use the tools is going to depend on the symptom you are treating. You may find your worst symptom is joint pain and not say, hot flushes, in which case you may find using the yoga and mindfulness tools more effective than say the breathwork. It is a matter of adapting and finding out which one works for you the best.

Unfortunately, we are limited in book format to demonstrate yoga, hypnosis, and breathwork, but I have laid out a plan in writing for the yoga and breathing exercises to be performed. The online programme has all of this in video, audio, and written format.

BREATHWORK

Paced Breathing and Pranayama for stress reduction

There are many types of breathing techniques, but we are focusing on Paced Breathing and Pranayama breathing here.

Breathing exercises are effective for stress reduction because they stimulate the vagus nerve which runs from your abdomen to your brain stem. This is part of the "rest and digest" Parasympathetic nervous system, as opposed to the Sympathetic nervous system responsible for "fight or flight" responses, manifesting as stress.

Triggering the parasympathetic nervous system calms you down, slows your heart rate, and allows you to feel better, think rationally and most importantly over time, build resilience. Stress is the common denominator in flushes, anxiety, and heightening pain.

Our bodies' physiological responses to changes in breathing can impact our feelings and thoughts, which in turn affects our physical symptoms and behaviours.

Pranayama (practise for 10-15 minutes)

"Prana," which means both breath and energy, is part of a set of breathing techniques known as "Prana-Yama" (the retention and rising/expanding of breath) which aims to directly influence one or more respiratory parameters (such as frequency, depth, and inspiration/expiration (in and out) ratio).

Pranayama, is yogic breathing that can help reduce stress and promote overall well-being. Here's a step-by-step guide for practising Alternate Nostril Breathing, which is a pranayama technique often used for stress reduction:

Alternate Nostril Breathing

1 Sit Comfortably:
Find a comfortable and quiet place to sit with your spine straight. You can sit on the floor with crossed legs or on a chair with your feet flat on the ground. Rest your hands on your knees in a comfortable position.

2. Relax Your Shoulders:
Allow your shoulders to relax and your face to soften. Close your eyes gently if you're comfortable doing so.

3. Prepare Your Left Hand:
Place your left hand on your left knee with the palm facing upward. This is known as the "Gyan Mudra" hand position.

4. Use Your Right Thumb:
Use your right thumb to close your right nostril and your right ring finger to close your left nostril. Your right index and middle fingers can rest lightly on your forehead or between your eyebrows.

5. Begin by Closing the Right Nostril:
Close your right nostril with your right thumb and inhale slowly and deeply through your left nostril. Fill your lungs with air.

6. Switch to the Left Nostril:
After inhaling, close your left nostril with your right ring finger, release your right nostril, and exhale completely through your right nostril.

7. Inhale through the Right Nostril:
Keeping your left nostril closed, inhale slowly and deeply through your right nostril.

8. Switch to the Right Nostril:
After inhaling, close your right nostril with your right thumb, release your left nostril, and exhale completely through your left nostril.

9. Continue the Cycle:
This completes one cycle. Continue the pattern, alternating between inhaling and exhaling through each nostril. Inhale through one nostril, switch, exhale through the other nostril, and continue in this manner.

10. Maintain a Smooth and Gentle Breath:
Focus on maintaining smooth, controlled, and gentle breathing throughout the practise. The breath should be steady and without strain.

11. Complete the practise:
Continue for about 5-10 minutes or as long as feels comfortable. To finish, complete the cycle by ending with an exhale through your left nostril.

12. Observe the Effects:
After completing the practise, sit quietly for a moment with your eyes closed, observing the effects of the breathing exercise on your mind and body.

Important Note:
- If you feel dizzy or lightheaded at any time during the practise, return to normal breathing and discontinue the technique if necessary.

Practising this technique regularly can help balance the nervous system, reduce stress, and promote a sense of calmness. **As with any new exercise or breathing technique, it's advisable to consult with a healthcare professional first on your suitability, especially if you have pre-existing health conditions.**

Paced Breathing

(once mastered, use for a few minutes throughout the day)
Paced breathing is a slow, controlled breathing technique that involves breathing from the abdominal area rather than the chest. The idea is that you slowly breathe in for a count, hold it for another count (optional) then breathe out slowly for a certain count. This is also known as diaphragmatic breathing.

The beauty of this type of breathing technique is that, once mastered, it is transportable and can be discreetly done throughout your day.

This type of breathing also known as abdominal or diaphragmatic breathing, can be a very helpful technique to manage hot flashes. Here's a step-by-step guide on how to perform paced breathing:

1. Find a Comfortable Position: Sit or lie down in a comfortable and quiet space. Ensure that your back is straight, and your shoulders are relaxed. You can close your eyes if it helps you focus.

2. Place one hand on your chest and the other on your abdomen, just below your ribcage. This allows you to feel the movement of your breath.

3. Inhale slowly and deeply through your nose. Focus on filling your lungs with air, allowing your abdomen to expand as you

breathe in. Your chest should rise only slightly, and the majority of the breath should be taken into your abdomen.

4. Once you've inhaled fully, pause for a brief moment. Hold your breath for a count of one or two. This pause is not a breath-holding exercise but a moment to focus on your breath.

5. Exhale slowly and completely through your mouth. Focus on emptying your lungs and allowing your abdomen to contract as you breathe out. The exhalation should take longer than the inhalation.

6. After you've exhaled completely, pause for another moment before starting the next inhalation. This pause helps to create a rhythmic and controlled breathing pattern.

7. Continue the cycle of slow, deep inhalations and complete exhalations. Aim for a comfortable and natural rhythm. You might start with a 4-4-4 count (inhale for a count of 4, hold for 4, exhale for 4) and adjust as needed.

8. As you practise paced breathing, bring your attention to the sensation of your breath. Pay attention to the rise and fall of your abdomen and the flow of air in and out of your body.

When you experience a hot flush, try to engage in paced breathing. Focus on the breath to promote relaxation and reduce the intensity of the hot flush. The flush will come and go but the intensity of it will be counteracted by the relaxation of the breathing.

Once you get the hang of this technique you can take this anywhere with you. You no longer need to sit or lie down or place your hands on the chest and abdomen. You are already aware of your breathing and the counting that goes with it. You could quietly stand, say in a meeting, and just practise this with your lips pursed so it's discreet and only you know that you're doing it; practise in a mirror first to see your expression then modify your lips until the technique looks and feels seamless and natural to you.

The goal is to create a relaxed and controlled breathing pattern. Paced breathing can be a valuable tool for managing stress and hot flushes, but individual experiences may vary. **It's advisable to consult with a healthcare professional for personalised guidance and to ensure that paced breathing is suitable for you specifically.**

YOGA

I'm sure by now you are well aware of the benefits of yoga. In this case, we are using the technique to alleviate joint pain. **Always check that you are physically fit to perform the exercises for example, it may not be suitable for patients with osteopenia or osteoporosis.**

Here's a 15-minute yoga sequence that targets both the upper and lower parts of the body, focusing on gentle movements to help alleviate joint pain. This sequence covers various joints, including shoulders, wrists, hips, knees, and ankles. Remember to listen to your body, move slowly, and breathe deeply. If you have any existing health concerns or conditions, it's advisable to consult with a healthcare professional before starting a new exercise routine.

Each exercise is to be done for approximately 2-3 minutes

Starting Pose-Easy Seated Pose (2 minutes):
- Sit comfortably with your legs crossed (if you can, otherwise sit on a chair)
- Rest your hands on your knees.
- Close your eyes and take deep breaths to centre yourself.

Neck and Shoulder Rolls (2 minutes):
- Inhale as you gently roll your shoulders up towards your ears.
- Exhale as you roll them back and down.
- Repeat this movement for 1 minute and then reverse the direction for another minute.

Wrist Exercises (2 minutes):
- Extend your arms in front of you.
- Circle your wrists in one direction for 1 minute and then switch to the other direction for another minute.

Cat-Cow Stretch (3 minutes):

Before   After

- Come onto your hands and knees in an all fours, tabletop position.
- Inhale, arch your back, and lift your head for Cow Pose.
- Exhale, round your back, and tuck your chin for Cat Pose.
- Repeat for 3 minutes, syncing the movement with your breath.

Downward Dog with Pedal (2 minutes):

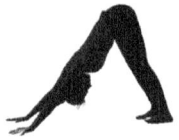

- Again from from tabletop position on all fours, lift your hips upwards and straightens your legs. You should look line an upside down V shape looking downwards
- Pedal your feet, bending one knee at a time to stretch the calves and hamstrings.
- Hold each stretch for a breath.

Chair Pose (2 minutes):

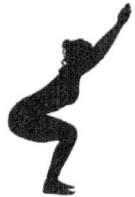

- Stand with feet hip-width apart.
- Inhale, raise your arms overhead, and bend your knees, lowering your hips into a seated position, move down to this position as far as you can
- Hold for a minute, breathing deeply.

Warrior II Pose (2 minutes per side):

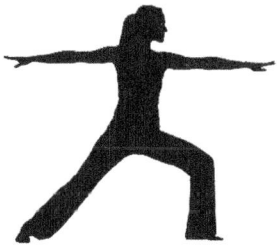

- Step one foot back, keeping the front knee bent.
- Extend your arms parallel to the floor.
- Hold for 2 minutes on each side.

Tree Pose (2 minutes per leg):

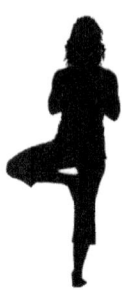

- Shift your weight onto one leg and bring the sole of the other foot to the inner thigh or calf.
- Bring your palms together in front of your chest.
- Hold for 2 minutes on each leg.

Seated Forward Bend (2 minutes):

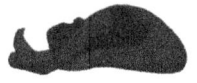

- Sit with your legs extended in front.
- Inhale, lengthen your spine, and exhale, hinge at your hips to reach forward.
- Hold for 2 minutes.

Legs Up the Wall (1 minute):

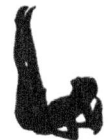

- Sit close to a wall and swing your legs up.
- Rest in this gentle inversion for 1 minute, focusing on deep breaths.

Final Relaxation-(1 minute):

- Lie on your back with legs extended and arms by your sides.
- Close your eyes, relax, and focus on your breath for 1 minute.

This sequence aims to gently stretch and strengthen the body, improving joint mobility and relieving stiffness. Adjust the duration of each pose based on your comfort level and gradually increase as your flexibility improves. **Always consult with a healthcare professional before starting any new exercise routine, especially if you have joint concerns or other health conditions.**

FOCUSED MINDFULNESS
(FOR BRAIN FOG + PAIN RELIEF)

Mindfulness is a mental state achieved by focusing your awareness on the present moment while calmly acknowledging and accepting your feelings, thoughts, and bodily sensations without judgement. It's almost like a meditation state. So here we are trying to concentrate all your focus on one thing and not be distracted, this will help in brain fog when you're trying to think or remember one thing.

Practising mindfulness or meditation for a few minutes (or for as long as possible) a day can strengthen areas of the brain responsible for memory, learning, attention, and self-awareness, and help calm down the sympathetic nervous system, ultimately improving cognitive function and clarity of thought.

This is a very simple but effective practise, here's how to do it:

"Find a comfortable position and gently close your eyes. Take a few deep breaths, allowing your body to relax with each exhale. Now, bring your attention to the sensation of your breath as it enters and leaves your body. Notice the rise and fall of your chest or the sensation of air passing through your nostrils. If your mind starts to wander, simply acknowledge the thoughts and gently bring your focus back to your breath. Continue this practise for a few minutes, allowing yourself to be fully present in the moment. When you're ready, slowly open your eyes and take this mindfulness with you as you continue your day"

Remember you are concentrating all your efforts on one thing, so it will take a little practise to master. This practise is designed to improve your focus and concentration with regular use.

For Pain Relief

By focusing on different body parts and acknowledging any pain or discomfort, you can develop a mindful awareness of your bodily sensations and potentially relieve tension.

Here's a short body scan mindfulness script for joint pain relief:

"Find a comfortable position, either sitting or lying down. Close your eyes or maintain a soft gaze. Take a few deep breaths, inhaling through your nose and exhaling through your mouth. Allow your body to relax with each exhale.

Now, bring your attention to your toes. Notice any sensations, including pain or discomfort. Breathe into these sensations, acknowledging them without judgment. Gradually move your focus up to your feet, ankles, and then your lower legs. Continue to observe any sensations and breathe into them.

Slowly shift your attention to your knees, thighs, and hips. Observe any sensations in these areas, and gently breathe into them. Allow your body to relax further with each exhale.

Move your focus to your lower back, abdomen, and chest. Notice any sensations and breathe into them, allowing your body to release tension. Continue to your upper back, shoulders, and neck, observing any sensations and breathing into them.

Finally, bring your attention to your arms, elbows, wrists, and hands. Notice any sensations and breathe into them. Conclude by focusing on your head and face, observing any sensations, and breathing into them.

Take a few more deep breaths, and when you're ready, gently open your eyes"

Remember the longer you practise the greater the benefit.

PELVIC FLOOR EXERCISE
(KEGEL EXERCISES)

Pelvic floor exercises, also known as Kegel exercises, can be beneficial for menopausal women to improve pelvic floor muscle strength and alleviate symptoms such as urinary incontinence, pelvic organ prolapse, and sexual dysfunction. This section is an introductory guide and needs to be worked through with a suitable health professional.

Millions of people across the world struggle with bladder weakness and stress incontinence.

As if menopause is not bad enough, pelvic floor weakness can have a dramatic effect on people's general quality of life as well as their physical and mental well-being.

The signs of bladder weakness can get worse with time if left untreated. However, all is not lost.

As with any other form of exercise, frequent pelvic floor exercises will strengthen the muscles over time, so they become more effective and provide the correct amount of support to the bladder to ensure leaks don't occur.

Additionally, it can soothe 'overactive' nerves in people who have irritable bladder feelings.

Please note, I am not a Physiotherapist so it is important to consult with a healthcare professional for an accurate diagnosis, safety, and personalised advice regarding bladder leakage triggers and management.

Whilst it is out of my scope of practice, Physiotherapists or an appropriately qualified individual, **may,** recommend the following steps to perform pelvic floor Kegel exercises:

1. Identify the pelvic floor muscles: Before starting the exercises, it's essential to locate the pelvic floor muscles. One way to do this is to imagine stopping the flow of urine midstream. The muscles you engage to do this are the pelvic floor muscles.

2. Find the right position: You can perform pelvic floor exercises in various positions, such as lying down, sitting, or standing. Choose a position where you feel comfortable and can focus on contracting the pelvic floor muscles effectively.

3. Start with relaxation: Begin by relaxing your pelvic floor muscles to ensure you're not already tensing them. Take a few deep breaths and allow your muscles to relax fully.

4. Contract the pelvic floor muscles: Once relaxed, contract your pelvic floor muscles by squeezing and lifting them. Imagine pulling them up and in as if you're trying to lift something using only your pelvic floor. Here is the important part, avoid tensing the abdomen, buttocks, or thigh muscles during the exercise.

5. Hold the contraction: Once you've contracted your pelvic floor muscles, hold the contraction for a few seconds, aiming for 5 to 10 seconds initially. Gradually increase the duration as your muscles get stronger.

6. Release and rest: After holding the contraction, release the pelvic floor muscles and allow them to relax completely. Take a brief rest period before starting the next repetition.

7. Repeat and progress: There is no "one size fits all" approach here. Our online therapist Tara recommends repeating the exercises no more than three times a day as a maximum.

As your pelvic floor muscles become stronger, gradually increase the number of repetitions and the duration of each contraction. The great thing about these exercises is that they can be done discretely with no gym membership or buying clothing etc. (American College of Obstetricians and Gynaecologists 2020, Dumoulin, C., & Hay-Smith, J. 2010)

It's important to note that it may take time to notice improvements, and consistency is key. The above is only a beginner's guide.

Working with a physiotherapist who specialises in pelvic floor rehabilitation can provide personalised guidance and ensure you're performing the exercises correctly and safely.

IMPORTANT

Please do not perform these exercises if you suffer any kind of pain, during urination, with an overactive pelvic floor, or any pelvic floor dysfunction. If you are not sure please seek advice from a suitably qualified health practitioner.

COGNITIVE BEHAVIOURAL THERAPY

The number of thoughts and emotions we have on a daily basis wildly fluctuate in number and can run into the thousands. Our thoughts tend towards a negative bias; this has been suggested because we tend to pay attention, learn from and make decisions based on negative information than positive ones. This maybe a protective mechanism hardwired into the brain. (Cacioppo et al. 2014)

Thoughts and emotions are interconnected and collectively contribute to the complexity of everyday behaviours. A thought can influence behaviour by interpreting situations, and guiding decision-making, whilst an emotion can serve as a motivator for behaviour for example fear may prompt avoidance or anger may lead to confrontation.

Cognitive Behavioural Therapy (CBT) is a widely practised form of psychotherapy that focuses on the connections between thoughts, feelings, and behaviours. This type of therapy helps to improve people's patterns of thinking and related behaviours. **It is not positive thinking**, but rather allows the person to modify their thoughts which then defines their daily experiences.

Pioneered by founding fathers Aaron T Beck and Albert Ellis in the 60's, this groundbreaking area of work is shown to be highly effective when practised on a daily basis.

I have been trained by the British Menopausal Society to use the therapy to help treat hot flushes and night sweats. This has been mainly based around the work of the following researchers and they should be credited here:

Green, S. M., E. Haber, R. E. McCabe, and C. N. Soares. 2010. "Cognitive-Behavioural Group Treatment (CBGT) for Menopausal Symptoms: A Pilot Study." Paper presented at the Association for Behavioural and Cognitive Therapies, San Francisco, November.

Diagnosis and management of menopause: summary of NICE guidance (2019)

Hunter MS, Chilcot J. Is cognitive behaviour therapy an effective option for women who have troublesome menopausal symptoms? Br J Health Psychol. 2021 Sep;26(3):697-708. doi: 10.1111/bjhp.12543. Epub 2021 Jun 8. PMID: 34101946; PMCID: PMC8453849.

The CBT Cycle

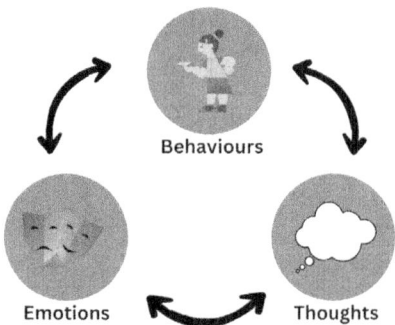

Figure 13: The CBT cycle

The fundamental idea behind CBT is that our thoughts, feelings, and behaviours are interconnected. A situation (trigger) creates certain thoughts and feelings which lead us to have a certain outcome i.e., the behaviour. Modification of thoughts then influences how we feel and ultimately how we respond to that situation.

The great thing about this therapy is that it focuses on the now and not the past. It is mainly concerned with the thoughts, emotions, and behaviours of the present-day problems you may be facing. So in the context of menopause, CBT focuses on the immediate issues which in this case are hot flushes and related anxiety.

CBT then breaks down unhelpful thoughts and negative feelings into more positive and realistic ones. In turn, our physical reactions and behaviours are then impacted by more positive outcomes.

As we will see later on in the action section, the therapy relies upon you monitoring your thought patterns and questioning yourself.

Because the cycle is connected, changing any one component affects the other which is why in the action section we will look to actively modify your behaviours to reduce the creation of triggers, but more on that later.

In this case, we are going to use CBT to change how you view your flush and sweat symptoms which will then affect how to respond and manage the issue

So we are going to break that habit cycle of unhelpful thoughts, so it will take a little effort and practise.

Let's take an example:

Meet Priya

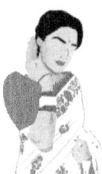

Priya enjoyed socialising but during menopause, she found the sudden arrival of a hot flush quite embarrassing and felt self-conscious about them. She started to avoid social gatherings and nights out as she felt that other people might notice.

Her thoughts included statements such as "god this is going to last forever" and "I will never be able to socialise again". Her worry and anxiety consumed her to the point that it disrupted her ability to socialise, talk to others and generally relax and have a nice evening out.

Meet Sarah

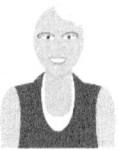

Sarah on the other hand also experienced unexpected hot flushes that made her uncomfortable, but she knew such an event would pass and most people didn't notice anyway and for those that did, she would just make a light-hearted comment around the matter.

She was prepared and would carry some wipes in her purse for just such an event, she was determined that it wasn't going to ruin her life.

You can see that both women experienced the same event i.e.,. a hot flush.

Both were aware of the uncomfortable nature of the problem, however the way each of them interpreted the situation and the resulting experience from, it was quite different.

Priya's interpretation led her to have negative thoughts and anxiety around the experience; "What will people think of me" and "I feel so embarrassed" were some of the thoughts that plagued her leading her to socially withdraw and have negative feelings around the matter.

Sarah, on the other hand, had a different viewpoint on the matter, she knew the flush was only going to be temporary and was it not the end of the world, she was already prepared and her thoughts and behaviours reflected that which led her to have a much better experience around the flush.

Because she had wipes on hand she felt more confident in her ability to deal with the situation and her thoughts of "this is not going to ruin my life" kept her patient, strong, and confident as the flush came and went. She continued to enjoy the evening with minimal disruption.

It should be noted at this point that Anxiety and Flushes go hand in hand here because of the similarity in symptoms.

Both cause a physical sensation of overheating, both lead to increased arousal and embarrassment and both cause avoidance-style behaviours.

CBT allows us to step back and understand the power that we have over how we respond to our daily challenges and is highly effective for anxiety and depression states.

Here CBT provides a framework that allows women to have greater coping mechanisms for their daily exposure of symptoms and experiences. This means a reduction of stress and anxiety as well as the intensity and number of hot flushes with daily practise.

Let's have a look at thought patterns and how they are affecting you daily.

Thought Distortions

As mentioned previously It is estimated that our number of thoughts runs into the thousands. These thoughts tend towards a negative bias and are repetitive from the previous day.

Thoughts can be influenced by various factors, such as our environment, previous experiences, cultural and societal influences, genetics, and even our current emotional and physiological states.

Nerves in the brain form intricate networks and pathways, and the patterns of activity within these networks give rise to the thoughts and mental processes we experience.

Both Albert Ellis and Aaron T Beck were pioneers in Behavioural Therapy. Ellis was involved in developing Rational Emotive Therapy in the 1990s, whilst Beck deduced the link between thoughts and feelings and also added the term cognitive therapy to the process. The Beck Institute stands today as an international authority on CBT research and resources.

David Burns in the 1980's listed a number of thought distortions also known as cognitive distortions. The work suggests that by correcting these distortions, a more realistic experience of events is then created. (Burns, D. D. 1980)

Example distortions include: (not exhaustive list)

Jumping to Conclusions: where you assume that a negative assumption has been made about you (also called mind reading) e.g., I must look terrible after a hot flush.

All or nothing patterns of thinking: Also called Black or White Thinking, this type of distortion leads you to think it's either one way or the other and nothing in between e.g., I will never sleep again.

Personalisation: where you negatively judge yourself or you attribute the negative feelings of others around you e.g., my husband is upset, it must be my fault.

Emotional Reasoning: when personal feelings are accepted as facts rather than reality e.g., I'm feeling inadequate, so I must be worthless.

Catastrophizing: is when someone assumes that the worst will happen e.g., If my boss sees me having another hot flush again I will get fired.

Should Statements: where you have high expectations of what you or other people should be doing or behaving e.g., I should have spent more time on that assignment.

Global Labelling: Global labelling occurs when we allow one particular trait or aspect of a person's behaviour to colour their entire character e.g., Priya is not coming out tonight, she must be a recluse.

Blaming: where we commonly hold either someone else or themselves responsible for the problem e.g., it's my boss's fault that I get stressed out at work.

Filtering: where you pick out and either minimise or magnify a particular event e.g., brushing off high praise from your boss as nothing (minimising) or "my argument with my husband this morning has ruined my entire day" (magnifying).

Fortune telling: When you predict events will unfold in a particular way e.g., I just know I'm going to get a hot flush at the restaurant tonight.

Overestimation of probability: You are overestimating the likelihood that an event will occur rather than it actually occurring e.g., I can never go out again.

We spend most of our lives just "thinking" rather than "categorising" as above.

However, just by being aware of the types of thought we have on a day-to-day basis, we have the ability to modify them to more realistic ones based on the events that have triggered them. As thoughts create our reality, the latter will also change as we modify our thoughts.

Priya

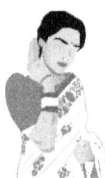

Let's look at Priya's thoughts again, they were all consuming to the point she couldn't socialise as she would have liked. Her statements included:

"god this is going to last forever" (Catastrophizing)
"I will never be able to socialise again" (Overestimation of probability)

"what will people think of me" (Personalisation/Global Labelling)
"I feel so embarrassed" (Personalisation)

Looking at the thoughts above we can see how unhelpful these are.

So Priya's automatic thought of "god this is going to last forever" is clearly out of proportion with reality. Nothing lasts forever.

But, at that point in time, it does create her reality, her feelings, her physical sensations, and eventually her withdrawal behaviour.

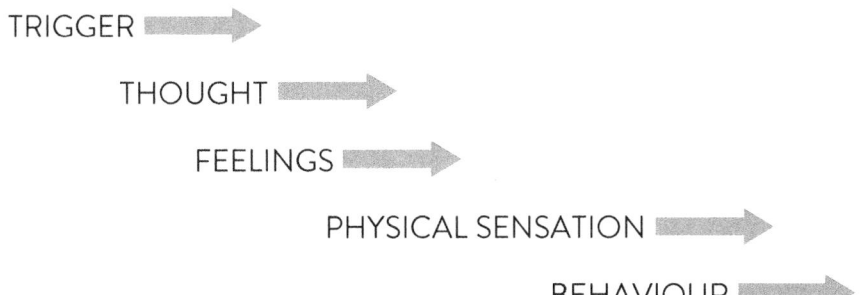

TRIGGER ➡

    THOUGHT ➡

        FEELINGS ➡

           PHYSICAL SENSATION ➡

                BEHAVIOUR ➡

In the CBT Model, The thoughts, behaviours, feelings, and physical sensations are all inter-connected, the negative cycles of thought that has been triggered can be interrupted and modified by changing our ways of thinking and the behavioural doing.

Understand here that the flush is coming as a result of physiological changes in the body and so you may not be able to predict when and where. So the goal would be to tone down the symptom's intensity as well as the anxiety and interference that the flush causes rather than to completely remove it. Likely you may not control the situation you find yourself in but you can modify how you think and feel about it.

Sarah

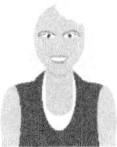

So looking at Sarah again,

Flush Trigger

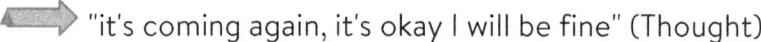 "it's coming again, it's okay I will be fine" (Thought)

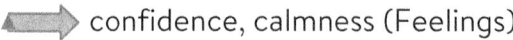 confidence, calmness (Feelings)

slight to moderate discomfort (Physical Sensation)

carries on as normal (Behaviour)

You can see here how Sarah's thoughts are more empathetic towards herself. She knows she will have an issue but she's ready and understands the fleeting nature of the problem, and only sees it that way. This is reflected in her stoic thought patterns; she will not be beaten by the event.

This allows her to cope more readily, alleviating the anxiety and pressure on herself. The flush has still come and gone but, because she thinks differently to the event, it has a different impact on her behaviour and her interpretation of the event compared to Priya.

Each of the components of the CBT cycle are linked, such that if one part is influenced, then it has a knock on effect to the other.

For example if an emotional sign such as worry was escalated to a full blown panic attack, then the initial physical sensation of the worry such such as a raised heart rate can quickly move up to a racing heart, thumping in the chest accompanied by a cold sweaty feeling i.e., the panic attack.

The reverse is also true, a racing heart can be calmed down to an eventually normal rate by having calming thoughts, strategic breathing techniques, behaviours of using a fan or drinking cool water etc., which means the associated anxiety is also de-escalated in its intensity.

Now that you understand the theory behind CBT, we will explore how to incorporate it into everyday practise when we treat hot flushes and night sweats later on. Please go through the CBT theory again if you need to.

YOUR ACTION
ROADMAP

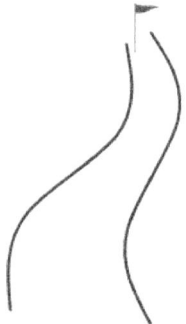

When trying to do or change anything in your life, the first step is the most difficult, because it frightens people. It's the one that denotes change, and change may be scary!

We feel at ease where we are because we know where we are and what to expect, in other words, we are in our comfort zone.

Taking the first step means doing something new and unfamiliar where things may not turn out as expected or planned. It means coming out of your comfort zone and experiencing discomfort.

However, as you are already in discomfort with your menopausal symptoms, by starting and continuing this programme you are in effect moving into a comfort zone where your issues start to improve.

So just like going to the gym, to maximise the benefits of this programme, you will need to set aside time each day to work through it.

There is a saying that goes "If you fail to plan then you plan to fail"

So Let's start planning. You could do this any way you choose, it's whatever works for you.

My suggestion is that you split your day into 3 main time zones

Morning before Work

The main part of the day

And The Evening

Now decide which tool you are going to use and in which time zone. For example, use Yoga during the morning when you have a spare 15 minutes. Then make sure you are monitoring your progress.

Cognitive Behavioural Therapy (CBT) is going to take a little bit of practise to master but this is potentially life-changing when done correctly, so please read and understand the module before you start attempting it. When you get the idea behind it, you can practise this at any time of the day because it revolves around thought patterns which you do all day anyway.

Now It doesn't matter how you use the tools as long as you use them. And use them as frequently as possible. Schedule the times of day with the least amount of distractions and the most amount of "me " time.

If you have a male partner, get them to read the book especially the section for men. It will be a long-term investment for them as well.

Each of the exercises is in effect, a little bit of homework! They are there for you to complete.

Find what works for you and stick to it. This programme is meant to be a holistic approach to your issues and you may find some areas may have more of an impact than others. So it will be a bit of a trial-and-error approach to see what is working.

Please give yourself at least 21 continuous days of practise when you use a particular tool. It's the repetitive suggestions that the mind and body will take on board, however this will only happen over time.

The more you practise the strategies here, the greater benefit you will experience daily as well as the improvement in quality of life. Remember the power is in your hands to change your day to day reality.

So let's begin by looking at the Action Roadmap. We will do a summary first, and then explore the roadmap in detail. You can create your own and adjust it for your lifestyle, this is only a suggested one. We are starting on the flushes. Give yourself 4-6 weeks of action-taking, monitoring and adjusting.

Action Roadmap Summary

I suggest you **start** this programme on **the weekend before Week 1**. I am also assuming you are not working on these 2 days.

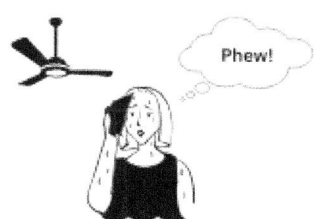

HOT FLUSHES, NIGHT SWEATS AND POOR SLEEP

Saturday Day 1 Sunday Day 2	• Explore top 3 issues, start morning tool(am), read CBT module • Complete Exercise 1 Disruption Sheet on Day 2 • Use am tool, Use pm tool
Week 1 Monday-Friday	• Am tool + Pm tool each day • Complete and Action Removing Triggers
Saturday Sunday	• Am and pm tool + Reflection on Week + Go through CBT Module again as a refresher • Am and pm tool + Review Exercise 1 (from Day 2) + start Re-framing Sheet
Weeks 2-4 Monday-Sunday	• Am tool+ Pm tool each day • Actively Remove Physical Triggers (ongoing) • Continue with CBT Re-framing Exercise
Weekend before Week 4 Saturday Sunday	• Reflect and Review Disruption sheet from Day 2 • Start Sleep Module and Menopausal Sleep Diary (Pm Tool is now the Sleep Hypnosis)

Weeks 4-6 Monday-Sunday	• Am tool+ Pm tool each day • Change triggers for poor sleeping • Continue practising CBT and Re-framing at every point
WEEK 6	REFLECT, REVIEW AND MODIFY, start new Issue e.g. Joint Pain

Here is the same table left blank in case you want to create your own plan

Reflection and starting weekend before Week 1 Saturday Day 1 Sunday Day 2	
Week 1 Monday-Friday	
Saturday Sunday	
Week 2 and 3 Monday-Sunday	
Weekend Before Week 4 Saturday Sunday	
Weeks 4-6 Monday-Sunday	
WEEK 6	

Action Roadmap in Detail

Weeks 1-2: Reflection and Starting

Reflection: Weekend before Week 1 or any 2 days off before starting the programme.

Day 1 Saturday before Week 1

Activities to do:

- Complete the Written Exercise below in the morning
- Start the morning with a tool
- Schedule in other relevant tool(s) to your issue and the time of day to be used

Exercise

Spend some time deciding which top 3 have the most impact on your daily life and you are going to tackle i.e., be Specific

If you have a partner then include them here in case they want to provide input.

Have a real deep down think about your worst symptoms of the programs that you can change

For example. 1 My flushes
2 My fatigue
3 My poor sleep

Symptom 1...

Symptom 2...

Symptom 3...

Now focus on **ONE symptom only**, to tackle
Don't make the mistake of trying to tackle all 3 at once!
Start with the worst, most problematic one first...

It is better to completely focus on one area at a time, this stops overwhelm and you are more likely to complete using small steps.

It's important to have measurable goals so that you can track your progress and stay motivated. Stay realistic in your goal. Look for small victories and not one huge one, it's the small ones that will keep you on track and stay motivated i.e., achievable.

For example when we tackle Hot Flushes:

You cannot cure the flush completely but you can reduce its intensity over time and how it is going to affect your life.

STARTING POINT: Goal Setting

Now that you have an idea of what you are going to tackle, It is important to set some sort of a goal....

The goal should move in a direction of achievement and not conclusion. For example "I want to improve my anxiety" and not "I want to stop worrying".

The key to any goal setting is to create **SMART** goals, this SMART acronym stands

for **S**pecific, **M**easurable, **A**chievable, **R**elevant, and **T**ime-bound.

It is a method of goal setting that helps individuals and organizations set clear, achievable objectives that increase the likelihood of success.

Here is a breakdown of what each letter in the SMART acronym stands for:

- Specific: Goals should be clear and specific, with a well-defined outcome.
- Measurable: Goals should be measurable, with specific criteria that can be used to track progress and determine success.
- Achievable: Goals should be achievable, taking into account available resources and skills.
- Relevant: Goals should be relevant to the overall mission or purpose of the organization or individual.
- Time-bound: Goals should be time-bound, with a specific deadline for completion.

Let's look at a goal as an example.

Set the goal of "I want to stop getting hot flushes"

This is too broad and a bit "wishy-washy." Let's look at this goal in a SMART way:

Make it Specific...so we are going to say "my aim is to reduce the intensity of flushes at work". Notice we have a directional goal and not a concluding goal.

Make it Measurable...so we are going to do this via recording in a diary or journal so you can see before and after results and if necessary quantify the number of flushes or their intensity.

Make Achievable...at this point, we need to be realistic about what we can achieve in a length of time, let's say reducing the number or intensity of flushes compared to normal.

Because there is no drug here to provide immediate benefit, It is the intensity and the thoughts and feelings around the event you are going to modify rather than expecting the flush to never appear. Be careful to be realistic in your expectations.

Make it Relevant... it is relevant because we want to reduce the discomfort in the workplace and generally feel better.

Make it Time-bound... so it will be achieved within "x" number of weeks.

You can see now how the initial ambiguous goal has more definition and structure. Now write down your goal.

My Goal is ....

After you have decided your number 1 problem area do the following **on the same day which is Day 1.**

Day 1
Morning: Start breathwork for stress reduction.

Tool Exercise

1. Take action! Schedule in and start practising now the paced breathing or pranayama breathing exercises to immediately reduce stress, preferably every morning. Note once the tools are incorporated into your life they are to be used every morning and evening.

2. On the same day, schedule when you are going to start any of the other tools you are going to use to tackle the issue at hand at different times of the day.

3. Evening: Re-read CBT Module

Day 1 is now complete

Day 2 (Sunday before Week 1)

Hot Flushes and Sweats Disruption

Tools to be used:

Breathing Exercises

1. Continue with morning Tool from Day 1 e.g., Pranayama

2. Complete the Exercise 1 Hot Flushes and Disruption Monitoring below and familiarise with hot flushes trigger reduction

3. Start another tool in the evening e.g., Paced Breathing or Hypnosis (online program only)

Have a starting point to see how the programme is making an impact over time. Use this example exercise and modify it to your main issue; here we are focusing on hot flushes and sweats.

Exercise 1: Hot Flushes Disruption Monitoring. This is a before, and after rating to see where you are before, and after doing this course.

Think back last week and answer the following:

How many hot flushes/night sweats did you have? (approximately)...............

How severe were they on a scale of 0-10 (circle)

0   1   2   3   4   5   6   7   8   9   10
none/mild   moderate   severe/unbearable

How much of a disruption did they make on your life a scale of 0-10 (circle)

0   1   2   3   4   5   6   7   8   9   10
none/mild   moderate   severe/unbearable

Important! List some of your exact thoughts by the words you use, your feelings and behaviours around these events (as many as you like), and then score them in terms of severity and disruption.

for example:

Situation or Time	Exact Thought Wording	Feelings	Behaviour	Severity 0-10 (how does it make you feel)	Disruption 0-10
Woke up at 3 am sweating	I'm never going to sleep	Frustrated Irritated	getting up	7	9

Table 1: Hot Flush Disruption Monitoring

This exercise is important as it is honing on how much disruption is being caused by your flushes or sweats and how you feel about it. The way you use your language is going to be important as you will see further on.

As you write things down see if things are happening on a regularity or any patterns may be emerging.

Hot flush/sweats trigger reduction.

Many people claim that when they are anxious or nervous, they experience hot flushes. The flight-or-fight response can be heightened by stress, and the adrenaline and cortisol rush that occurs when we perceive a threat may cause a hot flush. Flushes and sweats may well have common triggers but will be personal to you and your situation. Strong emotions, spicy foods, hot beverages, and heat itself, are all potential hot flush triggers.

Hot baths or wearing too much clothing can cause a hot flush, probably because they raise the body's core temperature, which expands the blood vessels. Other common triggers include alcohol, caffeine, medications, and disease states.

A pilot study found that participants who lost more than 10% of their body weight experienced a greater reduction in hot flushes than a control group. The study was published in Menopause: The Journal of the North American Menopause Society. The theory is that body fat is acting as an insulator. Therefore, it is more difficult to get rid of the heat from a hot flush, the more body fat you have. (Thurston et al. 2015)

Triggers for flushes can vary widely between women, with some not being able to particularly identify any at all. Others can include appliances that give off heat e.g., hairdryers, and certain fabrics like nylon or spandex which are less breathable.

Your ethnicity may also appears to play a role. In a study by Simpkins et.al, the findings indicated that African-American women experience hot flushes more frequently and with greater annoyance than women of other races. Caucasian women experienced fewer HFs per day than Hispanic women did. Whilst it's not known exactly why there are large variations in ethnicity triggers, it's probably genetics, diet, culture, environmental stressors, and/or socioeconomic status that would play some role in the ethnic differences in the expression and features of hot flushes. (Simpkins et al. 2009)

According to a study published in Maturitas: An International Journal of Midlife Health and Beyond, women who gave up smoking had fewer hot flushes overall, and fewer intensity and frequency than women who didn't, though it's unclear why smoking exacerbates hot flushes. (Smith et al. 2015)

Day 2 now complete

WEEK 1

Week 1 Monday-Friday

- Use morning and evening tools
- Complete Exercise 2: Removing Triggers below throughout the week

Exercise 2: Removing Triggers, involves creating a daily diary of situational events and triggers to both flushes and sweats. This should literally take you less than 30 seconds to complete. During your day you are looking out for triggers of your flushes. This will enable us to narrow down and focus on particular events and individual triggers of discomfort and what you could do to change them

Write down on a daily basis over the next week: Removing Triggers

Day of the week	Time of Day	The trigger e.g.,. smoking or seeing the boss or a physical place	What was triggered e.g., anxiety or racing heart, flush etc.	Distress level from 1-10 (1=low, 10=very high)	Changing Behaviour Action (start with easy small changes)	Reviewed Distress level (1=low, 10=very high)
Monday	10.30am	coffee	anxiety and racing heart	8	switched to de-caff	feel much less anxious probably a 3
Monday	7pm	wearing Lycra	gets me overly hot	7	switched to different fabric	2 definitely feel more comfortable

Table 2: Removing Triggers Monitoring

Weekend ending Week 1

Diary Reflection

Look back over the diary and ask yourself the following:

1. Can I immediately change any trigger factors? Or swap out any daily routines?

Yes. Priya changed her usual drive to work routine, she left 10 minutes earlier and took a slightly different route.

This new route had less traffic on it due to the side roads, which in turn reduced her anxiety about being on time. She now felt less hot and bothered about the whole situation. Reducing her anxiety meant reducing a risk of a hot flush before arriving at work. It was a good start to the day.

What can I change?

....

....

....

2. Did I notice any time of day that created the triggers, made them worse or better? What action could I take?

Yes. Sandra found Tuesday morning, after her boss received her weekly sales report, made her feel a lot calmer and less distressed about the report in general.

This reduced her anxiety and risk of getting a hot flush. She decided to explore why the report agitated her in the first place, and decided to take steps to remedy the situation and speak to her boss. This meant she counteracted her thought processes, and took action to see her boss. This small action paid off by reducing her weekly anxiety.

What action could I take?

....

....

....

3. Did certain events or situations made the triggers worse or better? Did I notice any patterns? What action could I take?

Yes. Emily noticed that going to the gym at her usual time made her feel self-conscious and ashamed of her body.

She felt a lot of eyes were glaring at her and that was creating unnecessary anxiety, making her feel hot and bothered. She decided to no longer put up with the situation and asked at the gym reception when the least busy periods were and if there were any female-only classes and instructors.

She felt very empowered by making the small but significant change. This immediately reduced the intensity of her anxiety and prevented any avoidance behaviours around going to the gym.

Did I notice anything, what could I change?

....

....

....

Over the next week period, you may see patterns emerging. Most people's lives are broadly similar and habitual on a day-to-day basis. We get up, go to work, come home eat and go to bed.

There may be certain triggers that you could immediately correct to reduce your discomfort e.g., changing gym gear to a lighter and cooler fabric or drinking a cold drink on your break instead of coffee. Others you may need to work on over several weeks for example certain stressors at work like members of staff or your boss, or finding the right bedding for ambient temperature.

A small amount of effort in writing a diary and making the subsequent changes will go a long way in helping you create a better quality of life for yourself.

- Carry on with morning and evening tools
- Go through the CBT Module
- Review Exercise 1 as mentioned below + Start Re-framing Sheet (Sunday)

By now you should have read through the CBT Module including the thought distortion categories and have completed Exercise 1 from Day 2 on Hot Flushes and Disruption Monitoring.

In Exercise 1 Hot Flushes and Disruption Monitoring, you looked back and identified some of your thoughts, feelings, and behaviours around the events that caused a hot flush or sweating episode and how it affected you.

Looking back at Exercise 1, see if your thoughts fall into any of the thought distortion categories.

Let remind ourselves of the categories and the exercise:

Jumping to Conclusions
All or nothing patterns of thinking
Personalisation
Emotional Reasoning
Catastrophizing
Should Statements
Global Labelling
Blaming
Filtering
Fortune telling
Overestimation of probability

Exercise 1

Situation or Time	Exact Thought Wording	Feelings	Behaviour	Severity 0-10 (how does it make you feel)	Disruption 0-10
Woke up at 3am sweating	I'm never going to sleep	Frustrated Irritated	getting up	7	9

Table 3: Hot Flushes and Disruption Monitoring Revisited

Your categorisation doesn't have to be accurate, you are not expected to be a therapist here!

At this point, you just need to be aware that you may be having a thought distortion that is affecting how you feel and behave, which may be unrealistic to the event caused.

Once you have identified a distortion, try to create a useful thought that is more realistic to the situation (the disruption may be minor but the thought may be out of proportion).

Here are a few examples of helpful thoughts or re-frames that may challenge your existing negative ones.

Am I being realistic about this?
Are there any advantages to continuing to hold this belief?
If my friend heard me say this, what would she say?
Is this helping me in any way?
I can do this, I have coping skills!
How would (name of someone you admire) cope with this?
This will pass, you got this!
What is the worst that could happen?
Is this forever or just now?

Test your thoughts, where is the supporting evidence that would back up your thought process? Look at the evidence now that would go against supporting the original negative automatic thought pattern.

This is a great exercise in helping you make decisions and changing certain beliefs whether they are core beliefs you have held or beliefs in the moment.

Here is an everyday example:

Trigger: My husband announces he's going away for a week on business

Your automatic thought: "He doesn't care about me, otherwise he would have told me earlier" or " Is he having an affair?"

Test your thought: Does he really not care? Is he really likely to be having an affair?

Where is the evidence to support both of these statements?

Re-examine and Reframe the thought: "This doesn't make any sense, he took me out for dinner Saturday night. I will quiz him and then I will check and get to the bottom of the situation".

Always test your thoughts, looking for the evidence in each case. In this case, he may well have just forgotten to mention it, or his boss may have sprung this upon him last minute. Always check the reality of the thought as this will allow you to put things into context and allow a basis for re-framing them.

Why your language matters

Early on in Exercise 1, I asked you to write down your thoughts in the exact words you would use. This is important to prevent you from labelling yourself as something you are not! In other words, distancing yourself from your thoughts and putting them into context.

Here's an example:

"I **am** a complete idiot for accepting that stressful position, it's making my flushes worse"

as opposed to

"I **feel** like a complete idiot for accepting that stressful position, it's making my flushes worse"

Note the slight but subtle shift in language between the 2 statements.

In the first "I am" statement, we are almost identifying ourselves as being an idiot. You are not an idiot, it's likely by now you will have raised a family and are juggling a career and partner. You may have made the occasional bad choice but on the whole, you are not a permanent idiot.

However, speaking thoughts this way almost identifies you in the negative statement.

Repeating statements of this type of nature can reinforce any negative core beliefs about yourself, so be aware of what language you use so that you can differentiate between who you are as a person and what you are thinking about.

In the second statement, "feeling like an idiot" is a transient state and likely to pass quickly. Nobody feels like an idiot constantly, just like nobody feels permanently happy or sad. This is a more forgiving statement.

Be mindful of your language and be more forgiving to yourself, this is part of the journey of reducing the intensity of the flushes and making them more acceptable in your life.

Practise Practise Practise!

It is important to practise consciously as if you are noticing your thoughts, feelings, and behaviours outside of your body. Imagine you are a friend who is then watching you. Your ability to make meaningful changes in your life will increase with your ability to take a step back, separate yourself from your problems, and identify the connections and differences between your actions, thoughts, and feelings.

Go back to Exercise 1 now and see if you can test and re-frame some of the thoughts you had in that exercise.

Thoughts from Exercise 1	Evidence favouring the thought	Evidence against supporting the thought	Type of Thought Distortion Experienced e.g., Personalisation	Useful, re-framed, helpful thoughts	How does the reframed thought feel in comparison to original thought? 0-10
God I'm so tired I will never go to to sleep again	I woke up automatically	Nobody never goes to sleep again!	All or Nothing	Yes I'm tired, but let's try again, sleep will eventually come	7 Yes i feel better, I'm tired but maybe I over-reacted
People think I'm unsociable	Because I never go out with people from work	Work Colleagues think I am unsociable That's because i don't like them. I love going out with my other real friends	Personalisation or Labelling	I do actually like going out and i will make more of an effort when I get my flushes under control	I feel better reviewing the thought, I think a 7 in this case

Table 4:Test and Reframe

I know I've thrown a lot at you, so to summarise. On the Saturday and Sunday ending of Week 1:

- diary reflection and trigger changes
- go through the CBT Model again
- Use Exercise 1 to start to try and identify the type of distorted thinking patterns you are generating during a flush or its anticipation
- Use Exercise 1 to start to reframe the thought in your favour being mindful of the language you say to yourself as well as putting the automatic thought into a reality context

PLUS: the morning and evening tools

Remember changing and challenging automatic negative thoughts is a habitual process and is going to take a little time, go easy on yourself and go for an 80/20 win scenario.

Weekend ending Week 1 Complete

WEEKS 2-4

Weeks 2-4 onward:

- Practise morning and evening tools
- Practise CBT module at every opportunity
- Keep a lookout for any triggers of flushes and change

Remember to review at the end of each week your progress and make changes. Being pro-active will be your saviour.

Over the next 2-4 weeks by practising CBT and using the other tools provided, you will strategically influence your thought and stress patterns to directly influence your behaviours and episodes of flushes and sweats.

Every negative thought will be counteracted by a positive one through habitual practise. You will begin to notice when a flush or sweat is arriving and start counteracting the thought; in time this will become second nature.

SUMMARY

By now you should have a clearer picture of your triggers, the level of disruption in your life, and what actions you can, or have already taken, to correct what you can correct. You should also be practising the tools daily and should by now notice a change compared to when you started.

With the hot flush triggers, start with small easy habits such as swapping a hot drink for a cold one or swapping out routines such as sitting under your normal desk to one under the air conditioning at work. Move over to the slightly more difficult tasks, ones like speaking to your boss about certain changes you would like to make during your workday when you feel more confident. Large changes such as stopping smoking should be approached with caution. You need to be in the right frame of mind and may need proper planning to take these on as failure may discourage you and set you back.

Then approach the CBT as a daily thought practise routine, always looking for the evidence and always re-framing the thought.

This programme is action-based. Only you can make these changes and only you will derive the benefit and empowerment from these changes. Build up your confidence on a day-to-day basis with the easy wins, stay focused and realistic as there always will be bad days, hey that's life!

But if you are winning 80% of the time you are absolutely on the path to changing the quality of your life. Allow yourself patience as this is a work in progress and please don't beat yourself up if you don't get immediate results, they will come.

Weekend before 4 weeks Review

- Review the disruption monitoring as below
- Start the Sleep Module if this was not your primary problem

After at least 4 weeks of continual practise please review the initial Disruption Sheet you completed on Day 2 of this programme.

Hot Flushes Disruption Monitoring...This is a before and after rating to see where you are before and after doing this course.

Now have a look at where you are in comparison to the original Exercise:

How many hot flushes/night sweats are you now having? (approximately)............

How severe are they on a scale of 0-10

0	1	2	3	4	5	6	7	8	9	10
none/mild					moderate			severe/unbearable		

How much of a disruption are they making on your life now on a scale of 0-10

0	1	2	3	4	5	6	7	8	9	10
none/mild					moderate			severe/unbearable		

How do you feel now

....

....

....

Are there areas you need to work on?

....

....

....

List how and when you are going to tackle these

....

....

....

This will be a bit of a to and fro exercise but persistence is key here and it will pay off.

Moving forward: Keep practising the relevant techniques provided.

Go back to the CBT training if you find yourself lapsing. Reflect and make changes in your life the SMART way, especially to keep a lid on stress.

Be bold and always be open to new practises to help manage your changes.

Remember if you are struggling, reach out for help. Think about speaking to health professionals, especially if they specialise in a particular area you are having trouble with.

You may need to add a low dose of medication or supplements just to take the edge off things. Be kind to yourself, and find "me time", this is an emotional roller-coaster and you may have a lot on your plate. Hopefully, you will have a supportive partner on your journey.

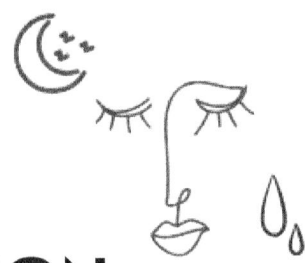

SLEEP DISRUPTION INCLUDING NIGHT SWEATS

Tools to be used:

Breathing Exercises
Sleep Diary and Hygiene
CBT
Yoga

Night sweats and flushes experience the same vasomotor symptoms in the body. The raising of temperature, the warmth and discomfort around the neck and chest area etc.

By now you should have a list of controllable triggers that could cause these physical symptoms.

Again change what you can control. Take a look at the following list of sleep disruption triggers and tips; implement them and see if they help:

- Avoid caffeine after noon midday. The length of time the body takes to break down the caffeine may disrupt sleep patterns.
- If you are on any medications then check with your pharmacist or doctor to see if they are disrupting your sleeping patterns. Also, be aware certain medical conditions such as Restless Leg Syndrome or Sleep Apnoea could also be affecting your sleep.
- Avoid other stimulants such as alcohol and nicotine for 4-6 hours before you go to bed.
- Avoid eating or late-night exercise for at least 3hrs before you go to bed.
- Avoid other artificial sleeping agents that hijack your natural chemicals needed to help you go to sleep e.g., over the counter sleeping tablets or antihistamines. Check with your Pharmacist.
- Napping can reduces the chemicals needed to stimulate sleep at night. Try and limit or completely avoid this activity where possible.
- The bedroom should be for sex and sleep only. Avoid screen time of any type, especially your phone which once again disrupts the natural sleep hormone Melatonin. Perhaps the only exception to this is listening to your hypnosis recording as you drift off to sleep.
- Look at your bedding. Do you need a new mattress or pillows? Do you need to change the duvet or blankets to a more cooling sheet? Do you need to change your pyjama fabric to cooler ones or sleep naked?
- Can you regulate the temperature of your bedroom environment? Can you open a window an hour before bed to cool the room down? Do you need an extra sheet on the bed in case you get chilly?

- Your body will naturally lower in temperature in the night as your metabolism slows down and your move less. If you are sleeping with a partner, consider extra blankets just for them so that they are not left in the cold. Can you keep a fan/air conditioning or cooling drinks/cold water bottles near your bedside?
- Is your lunch too heavy or too carb rich making you feel lethargic? Can you change anything here?
- Is eating spicy foods/hot drinks in the evening likely to trigger any flushing?
- If you have a partner, are they keeping you awake?
- Can you create a bedtime routine of switching everything off an hour before bed? This will help to wind you down and set the mood for sleep. If you combine this with a more regular eating and exercise pattern, this will be very helpful as the body likes routines. Lower the lighting which stimulates sleep.
- Use the breathing techniques available to you to lower your stress
- If overthinking is keeping you awake, write things down so thoughts go from your mind to paper. Worrying and anxiety further fuel worrying and anxiety and therefore are counterproductive. Could you discuss your anxious thoughts with someone before bed? Repeating or shouting your words out aloud also helps to release the thoughts from the mind.
- Use the 15-minute rule to try and remove the "forcing of sleep". Don't stay in bed if you still don't fall asleep after 15 minutes. Get up, go to another room, dim the lights, and try something dull, such as reading a boring book or an equally dull magazine. If a hot drink is not a trigger for flushing then have a non-caffeinated one to help you back in the sleep mode.

If after another 15 minutes you're still awake, get up again and continue the process until you feel sleepy. This promotes the association of your bed with slumber. Don't force sleep, it should come naturally as it does to all animals. Sometimes attempting to slumber prevents you from falling asleep.

Take away the struggle and anxiety associated with staying conscious. Just softly tell yourself, "I'll remain awake for a few more minutes and when I'm ready, I'll fall asleep naturally," rather than deliberately keeping yourself awake or scolding yourself for not being able to sleep.

Sleep is essential not only for rest and recuperation but for optimal mind and body functioning. It's another complicated area that involves chemicals, hormones, cycles, and rhythms and can be affected by many factors such as stress and trauma. This is why you can't just switch off like a light switch and suddenly go to sleep. How people sleep and their length also varies from person to person. You probably know of people who could sleep through an earthquake and others who would wake at the slightest noise.

There are two phases of sleep, Rapid Eye Movement (REM) and Non-Rapid Eye Movement (REM) sleep. The latter are then further subdivided into three stages, N1 N2, and N3. Each of these phases and stages involves changing in brain waves, eye movements, and muscle relaxation. The body goes through each step four to six times during one night, with each cycle lasting approximately 90 minutes. (Memar P et al. 2018). If you wake up naturally you are likely the end of a cycle. Waking during a cycle can leave you exhausted and irritable.

Research suggests hot flushes and night sweats that occurred during the second half of the night tended to happen due to either arousal or being woken up in the first half of the night. It appears REM impairs the thermoregulatory response, such as sweating and blood vessel dilation mechanisms, which may lead to the hot flush. (Freedman et al. 1992)

It is vital to try and do as much as you can to suppress the triggers that you can control to an absolute minimum. Creating a sleep diary will allow you to do that. This will be helpful not only for flushes, but also for anxiety, or any other cause of your insomnia/waking. Please fill in the sleep diary on the next page as part of the ongoing monitoring.

Menopausal Sleep Diary

	Weekly Notes And Triggers	Monday	Tuesday	Wednesday	Thursday	Friday	Saturday	Sunday
Complete during the night or early next morning	Time went to bed	9pm						
	Time woke up	2am						
	Reason for night time waking	too hot						
	Thoughts/ Images/Fe elings	irritated/ I will never sleep						
	Helpful Thoughts /Images/F eelings	I will change the blanket and it will be better						

Complete before going to bed	Hours actually slept	6						
	Time of exercise	5pm						
	Time of eating before bed	8pm						
	Alcohol consumed (number)	none						
	Caffeinate d drinks consumed (tea, coffee, fizzy drinks, chocolate based) (number and time)	11am and 4pm						
	Daytime nap? Y or N	N						

Table 5: Menopausal Sleep Diary

Having a diary like this will help you monitor your sleep patterns as well as any thoughts or images that may come up during the night. It will also allow you to review your triggers and quickly make changes where you can including your thoughts, for example going to the gym earlier at say 4 pm instead of 7 pm. We mentioned before to choose the language carefully as it matters.

Seize the moment and take action, it will only take a moment to fill. Use the diary over 1-2 weeks. The stress reduction tools will help you to cool your mind, and reduce your stress and all the internal hormones that go with that like cortisol and adrenaline.

Weeks 4-6: Monday to Sunday

Morning and Evening tools
Change the triggers for poor sleeping
practise CBT and re-framing at every point

Week 6 **REFLECT**: after 6 weeks of using the tools and making the relevant changes and monitoring, you should have noticed a significant improvement in your flushes and sleep patterns.

Now is the time to **REVIEW** what has worked and what needs further work for you to **MODIFY**.

If you are happy then time to look at a new symptom.

This now completes the Roadmap Action Plan for Hot Flushes, Night Sweats and Poor sleep

JOINT PAIN

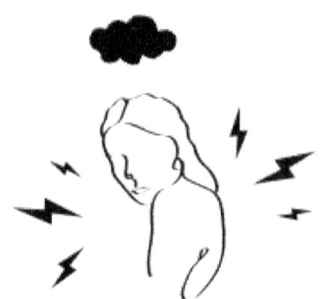

Tools to be used:

Mindfulness for Joint Pain
Yoga
Breathing Exercises
Eating Plan (Please see Eating For Menopause in the main part of the book)

There are a number of ways to help with joint pain, here we are using Yoga as part of mind-body techniques to help alleviate joint pain.

Yoga with an instructor combines physical postures, breathing exercises, and meditation. It improves joint flexibility, muscle strength, and reduces stress. Yoga has shown promising results in reducing joint pain and improving overall well-being. (Lauche et al. 2016)

Whilst there is no meditation here, please use the Mindfulness for Joint Pain and Breathwork as techniques to help reduce joint pain around the body.

If you have read Joint Pain in the main section of the book then you will understand that the pain comes from a stance of inflammation. An eating plan would be a way for you to introduce anti-inflammatory foods into your daily eating patterns to help combat pain and easing inflammation.

Although CBT can be helpful in this regard, we won't discuss it here because, regrettably, my training restricts me to hot flushes. Nonetheless, you can use the same concepts we previously covered to manage pain.

The Action Plan is:

Start Using Tools from Day 1
Change Trigger factors you can Control
Use Joint Pain Diary to monitor progression and the end of each week

My Goal is ....

Start by monitoring using the following Joint Pain Disruption Sheet: This is a before and after rating to see where you are before and after doing this course.

Think back last week and answer the following:

Rate the intensity of your joint pain on a scale of 0 to 10, with 0 being no pain and 10 being the worst pain imaginable.

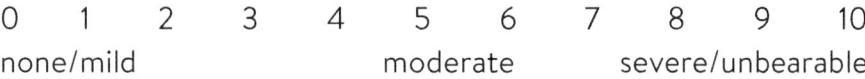

How much of a disruption does it make on your life a scale of 0-10

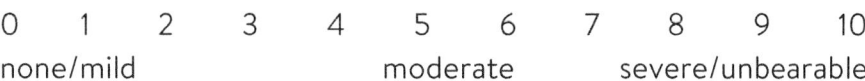

Important! List some of your exact thoughts by the words you use (this is important as you will see later),your feelings and behaviours around these events (as many as you like) and then score them in terms of severity and disruption. If you have already used CBT for hot flushes then you know about changing of the thoughts.

Situation	Exact Thought Wording	Feelings	Behaviour	Severity 0-10	Disruption 0-10
knee pain on stairs	I'm never going to get rid of this	despair	stopping, sitting, head in hands	7	9

Table 6: Joint Pain Disruption Monitoring

Joint Pain Roadmap

Reflection and starting weekend before Week 1 Saturday Day 1 Sunday Day 2	• Decide your goal for Joint Pain. • Complete disruption sheet • Start morning tool (am) • Am + Pm tools • Review Joint Pain Triggers Sheet including your regular diet
Week 1-4 (6) Monday-Friday	• Am and Pm tools daily • Daily monitoring and changing of triggers
Saturday and Sunday of each week	• Every weekend complete the reflection and review your progress making the changes for the following week
WEEK 4 or 6	• Review progress by going back to the Disruption Sheet you filled on Day 1

See the below monitoring sheet for you to complete everyday of each week. Remember to apply the 80/20 rule of winning we went through earlier in the book.

The monitoring is for you to complete every day when you get a moment, it's brief, but vital for you to identify trends or patterns so you can modify, and then review at the end of the week.

Joint Pain Diary

Weekly Notes And Triggers	Monday	Tuesday	Wednesday	Thursday	Friday	Saturday	Sunday
How did I sleep	Poorly						
Reason?	Shoulder Ache						
Action taken and Thought	irritated/ I will never sleep/ took painkiller						
Helpful Thoughts /Images/Feelings/actions	I will try and sleep in another position						
Weather	damp						

Complete during the night or early next morning

Complete before going to bed	Activities causing Pain	stair climbing							
	Medication /supplements taken? If so how much?	none this am							
	Type of Food or Drink contributing if any?	not							
	Is Mood/ Stress contributing?	not thought about it..hmm will consider							
	What Action am I going to take?	buy fish oil today							
	What Tools am I going to use?	Yoga							
	Effectiveness and modifications	Yes working							

Table 7: Joint Pain Diary

This is just a suggested diary. You can make your own monitoring diary, I have based the above table on the following information:

Activities:
- List the activities you engaged in during the day (e.g., walking, exercising, household chores, work related including stress).
- Note if any specific activities worsened or alleviated your joint pain.

Weather Conditions:
- Observe the weather conditions (e.g., temperature, humidity) and how they may have influenced your joint pain.

Dietary Factors:
- Document your food and drink intake.
- Identify any that seem to affect your joint pain positively or negatively.
- Consider the Mediterranean style of eating or at least reduce your sugar intake. Processed refined sugar is a huge contributor towards an inflammatory state, try and get it down or eliminate it completely if you can.

Medications and Supplements:
- Record any pain medications, over-the-counter remedies, or supplements you took to manage your joint pain.
- Note the dosage and time of administration.
Make sure you have adequate Vitamin D and Omega 3 fatty acids to alleviate joint inflammation.
Vitamin D, Fish Oils, Glucosamine, MSM, Chondroitin, Boswelia, Magnesium supplements are all useful to alleviate joint pain. I suggest you get proper clinical advice before buying.

Therapies and Treatments:
- Use the tools provided and see what impact they are making, alternatives could be acupuncture, heat and cold therapies, therapeutic massage.

General Well-being:
Sleep Quality:
- Rate the quality of your sleep on a scale of 1 to 5, with 1 being poor and 5 being excellent.
- Note if your joint pain affected your sleep patterns.

Mood and Stress Levels:
- Assess your mood and stress levels on a scale of 1 to 5, with 1 being low and 5 being high.
- Observe if there are any correlations between your mood, stress, and joint pain.

Patterns and Trends: Just like a pilot who makes adjustments before their plane lands, you too need to make the necessary adjustments.
- Look for patterns or trends in your joint pain experience over time.
- Note if certain triggers consistently worsen or alleviate your pain.

Progress and Improvement:
- Reflect on any changes or improvements in your joint pain symptoms.
- Celebrate small victories and milestones, and identify factors that contributed to positive changes.

Weekly Reflection

What worked, what didn't?

....

....

....

What am I going to change?

....

....

....

Did I do everything I planned?

....

....

....

If not why not, what stopped me and how can I change things?

....

....

....

Progress not perfection should be your mantra. Keep moving forward; you are here to change your life, which will unavoidably require some time and effort. It might take you a little longer than anticipated. You will get there!

Weeks 4-6 Review

Review your overall progress across the week and see how far you have come by filling in the Joint Pain Disruption Sheet:

Rate the intensity of your joint pain on a scale of 0 to 10, with 0 being no pain and 10 being the worst pain imaginable.

0   1   2   3   4   5   6   7   8   9   10
none/mild   moderate   severe/unbearable

How much of a disruption does it make on your life a scale of 0-10

0   1   2   3   4   5   6   7   8   9   10
none/mild   moderate   severe/unbearable

Now review the exact thought wordings you use daily. How have they changed from the initial sheet?

Situation	Exact Thought Wording	Feelings	Behaviour	Severity 0-10	Disruption 0-10
knee pain on stairs	I'm never going to get rid of this	despair	stopping, sitting, head in hands	7	9

Table 8: Joint Pain Disruption Revisited

This now completes the Roadmap Action Plan for Joint Pain.

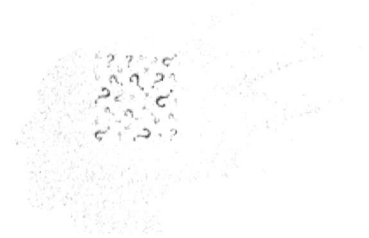

BRAIN FOG

Tools to be used:

Mindfulness Meditation
Yoga
Sleep Module (see Hot Flushes module)
Breathing Exercises
Eating Plan (see Eating for Menopause in the main part of the book)

Here's some food for thought in your brain fog journey:

Get Adequate Sleep: Prioritise 7-9 hours of quality sleep each night to support brain function, memory consolidation, and mental alertness. Do the Sleep Module if you haven't already.

Stay Hydrated: Drink plenty of water throughout the day to maintain proper brain function and prevent dehydration-related cognitive decline. Even mild dehydration can impair cognitive performance.

Balanced Diet: We all know this by now. Consume a nutrient-rich diet that includes fruits, vegetables, whole grains, healthy fats, and lean proteins. Aim to lower carbohydrates intake to no more than 100 grams per day where possible. Nutrients like omega-3 fatty acids, antioxidants, and B-vitamins have been associated with improved cognitive function.

Mindful Meditation: Use the mediation tool provided and engage in mindfulness meditation for a few minutes daily to reduce stress, enhance focus, and improve cognitive flexibility.

Regular Exercise: Incorporate short bursts of physical activity throughout the day to boost blood flow to the brain, promoting neuroplasticity and cognitive function. Exercise has been linked to enhanced memory and concentration. (Henriette van Praag 2009).

Limit Sugar and Processed Foods: This is a big one. Reduce consumption of sugary and processed foods, as they can cause fluctuations in blood sugar levels, leading to cognitive fog and reduced focus and general fatigue, think post lunch slump.

Prioritise Mental Breaks: Take short breaks during mentally demanding tasks to prevent mental fatigue and maintain cognitive clarity. Brief periods of rest improves focus and productivity.

Manage Stress: Employ stress-reduction techniques such as deep breathing, yoga, or progressive muscle relaxation to lower cortisol levels, which can negatively impact memory and concentration. (Vogel et al. 2016). Relaxation also reduces the movement of blood away from the brain for example in a stressful situation, which helps to maintain cognitive stability.

Limit Multitasking: Focus on one task at a time to enhance concentration and reduce cognitive overload. Multitasking can lead to reduced performance and increased brain fog. (Reference: The Myth of Multitasking – Psychology Today).

Brain-Boosting Supplements: Consider adding evidence-backed supplements like omega-3 fatty acids, vitamin D and ginkgo biloba to support brain health and reduce cognitive decline.

Cognitive Training: Engage in brain-training exercises or games designed to enhance memory, attention, and processing speed. These activities can help combat brain fog and cognitive decline.

Maintain Social Connections without Online Social Media: Regularly interact face to face with friends and family to stimulate the brain, improve mood, and reduce the risk of cognitive decline. Social engagement has been linked to cognitive resilience, however a slave to social media, emails etc. tends to lead to an attention exhaustion.

Optimise Vitamin B Levels: Adequate levels of B-vitamins, particularly B12 and folate, are essential for cognitive function. Consider supplementation if needed, as deficiencies can lead to brain fog. Check to see whether any medications are interfering with vital mineral absorption e.g., anti acid blockers inhibit the absorption of B12.

Limit Caffeine Intake: While moderate caffeine consumption can improve alertness, excessive intake can lead to jitters and decreased cognitive performance. Balance caffeine consumption to avoid brain fog, preferable no more than 2 per day before 12pm.

Practise Good Posture: Maintain proper posture to enhance blood flow to the brain and support spinal health, which can positively impact cognitive function. Slouching may lead to reduced oxygen flow and brain fog.

Reduce Screen Time: Not only does it suck you attention away from more important areas but prolonged excessive screen time can lead to eye strain, mental fatigue, and impaired cognitive performance.

Intermittent Fasting: Consider intermittent fasting, under medical supervision, as it has shown potential cognitive benefits through various mechanisms, including neuroplasticity. (Mattson et al. 2020).

Limit Alcohol Consumption: Moderation is key when consuming alcohol, as excessive alcohol intake can impair cognitive function, think of any wild night out!

Brain Games and Puzzles: Engage in intellectually stimulating activities like crossword puzzles, Sudoku, or chess to challenge the brain and improve cognitive function.

The Action Plan is:
Start Using Tools from Day 1
Change Trigger factors you can Control
Monitor progression and the end of each week

Roadmap

Reflection and starting weekend before Week 1 Saturday Day 1 Sunday Day 2	• Decide your goal for Brain Fog • Start morning tool (am) • Am + Pm tools • Review Brain Fog Triggers including your regular diet
Week 1-4 (6) Monday-Friday	• Am and Pm tools daily • Daily monitoring and changing of • triggers
Saturday and Sunday of each week	• Every weekend complete the Adjustment Diary and review your progress making the changes for the following week
WEEK 4 or 6	• Review progress by going back to the Initial Sheet you filled on Day 1

My Goal is ....

Start by monitoring using the following Brain Fog Disruption Sheet: This is a before and after rating to see where you are before and after doing this course

Think back last week and answer the following:

How bad is my Brain Fog on a scale of 0 to 10, with 0 being none and 10 being severe.

0	1	2	3	4	5	6	7	8	9	10
none/mild					moderate			severe/unbearable		

How much of a disruption does it make on your life a scale of 0-10

0	1	2	3	4	5	6	7	8	9	10
none/mild					moderate			severe/unbearable		

Important! List some of your exact thoughts by the words you use (this is important as you will see later),your feelings and behaviours around these events (as many as you like) and then score them in terms of severity and disruption.

If you have already used CBT for hot flushes then you know about changing of the thoughts

Situation	Exact Thought Wording	Feelings	Behaviour	Severity 0-10	Disruption 0-10
can's find my keys	aaaargh! not again	despair	stomping around angrily looking	8	9

Table 9: Brain Fog Disruption Monitoring

As part of the monitoring, we will look at a 3 step approach:

Step 1

Identify possible reasons where the brain fog maybe coming from.

Questions to ask yourself include:

1. How often do I experience brain fog? Is it a sporadic occurrence or a regular problem?
2. When does brain fog typically occur? Is it associated with certain activities, times of day, or specific triggers?
3. Am I getting enough sleep? Are there any disruptions to my sleep pattern?
4. How is my overall stress level? Am I managing stress effectively?
5. Have any recent changes in my diet or eating habits be affecting my cognitive function?
6. Am I staying hydrated throughout the day? Dehydration can contribute to brain fog.
7. Have I been exercising regularly? Physical activity can have a positive impact on mental clarity.
8. Are there any underlying health conditions or medications that might be causing or exacerbating brain fog?
9. Have I been exposed to any environmental toxins or allergens that could be affecting my cognitive function?
10. How is my mental health? Am I experiencing symptoms of anxiety, depression, or other mood disorders?
11. Have I been engaging in activities that stimulate my brain, such as reading, puzzles, or learning new skills?
12. Am I taking breaks and allowing myself time for relaxation and leisure activities?

13. Have I been socialising and maintaining meaningful connections with others?
14. Are there any specific thought patterns or negative self-talk that could be contributing to my brain fog?
15. Have I experienced any recent head injuries or concussions that might be affecting my cognition?
16. Have i started any new medications recently that maybe contributing? or any old ones that i didn't think about that maybe contributing?
17. 17 Have I looked at the obvious choices like overdoing alcohol, recreational drugs or pretty much overdoing anything?

Step 2

Monitor your daily patterns to see if you can identify where the brain fog is coming from. See if you can isolate it to the times of the day you get it the most. Note, if you have identified multiple reasons for your brain fog then only try and tackle them one at a time using the SMART goal system mentioned in the beginning of the programme

Here is a suggested 1-2 weeks diary that you could use, feel free to modify it based on your own circumstances

Brain Fog Diary

Time of the Day	Hours Slept (either total or fragmented)	Food and Drinks consumed	Approximate Hydration (ml) Aim for 2l/day	Activities done (at home/ at work)	Level of Stress/ Fatigue	Amount of Screen-time (min/hrs)	Brain Fog level (1-10)	Any relevant Notes
6-7 am								
7-8 am								
8-9 am								
9-10 am								
10-11 am								
11-12 am								
12-1 pm								
1-2 pm								
2-3 pm								
3-4 pm								

4-5 pm								
5-6 pm								
6-7 pm								
7-8 pm								
8-9 pm								
9-10 pm								
10-11 pm								
11-12 pm								
12-1 am								
1-2 am								
2-3 am								
3-4 am								
4-5 am								
5-6 am								

Table 10: Brain Fog Diary

Step 3

Once you have identified any issues, look at the obvious triggers to change and start to modify them one at a time and notice if they are having an effect on your brain fog.

Start with the easy ones initially for example drinking more water during the day and keep tabs on that, then move onto the ones that you feel require more of a behaviour change e.g., reduce excessive alcohol intake.

Adjustment Diary

Adjustments made in the following areas
Time of the Day Hours Slept Food and Drinks consumed Approximate Hydration (ml) Activities done Level of Stress/Fatigue Amount of Screen-time
Which Tools Used
New Brain Fog Level (1-10)
Relevant Notes What worked/didn't? What am I going to change?

Table 11: Adjustment Diary

As mentioned earlier, pilots make adjustments in flight before they can land at their destination. Please be the pilot here and forge ahead on until you find what works for you. This is an investment in your own improvement and well-being. It may take a little back and forth to see where you stand.

Weeks 4-6 Review

So as part of the progress, go back to the initial Brain Fog Disruption monitoring sheet and check to see how far you have come.

How bad is my Brain Fog on a scale of 0 to 10, with 0 being none and 10 being severe.

0	1	2	3	4	5	6	7	8	9	10
none/mild					moderate			severe/unbearable		

How much of a disruption does it make on your life a scale of 0-10

0	1	2	3	4	5	6	7	8	9	10
none/mild					moderate			severe/unbearable		

Now review the exact thought wordings you use daily. How have they changed from the initial sheet?

Situation	Exact Thought Wording	Feelings	Behaviour	Severity 0-10	Disruption 0-10
can's find my keys	aaaargh! not again	despair	stomping around angrily looking	8	9

Table 12: Brain Fog Disruption Monitoring Revisited

This concludes now the action plan and roadmap for treatment of Brain Fog

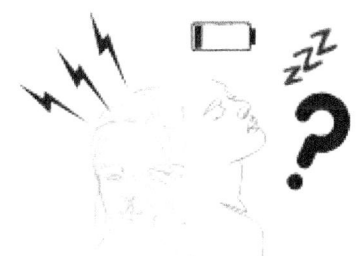

FATIGUE

Tools to be used:

Yoga
Breathing Exercises
Eating Plan
Mindfulness
Sleep Hygiene (see Hot Flushes module)

Menopausal Fatigue is often described as a lack of energy or constant exhaustion. This can range from mild to severe symptoms.

If we did a deep dive into cellular processes, fatigue is fundamentally a result of a lack of energy. There is insufficient energy available to the body to carry out its functions.

This is caused by an imbalance somewhere which is leading to the symptoms. In the case of menopause, symptoms range anywhere from brain fog and tiredness to depression and simply a lack of motivation to do anything. Symptoms can be short-lived or on an ongoing basis which may be described as Chronic Fatigue Syndrome or CFS.

Here our focus is Menopausal Fatigue which can be managed by lifestyle changes. Chronic fatigue syndrome (CFS), also known as Myalgic Encephalomyelitis, is a complex multi-system disease that is characterised by severe fatigue, cognitive dysfunction, sleep problems, dysfunction of the nervous system, and post-exertion malaise that severely impairs activities of daily living. This is beyond the scope of this book and needs to be investigated initially by your doctor. If this is affecting you, please don't hesitate to seek help.

If you think of the body as a battery, in theory, when you have woken up from a night's rest then your battery should be full of energy, ready to be used for the day. As your energy is used throughout the day the battery becomes drained waiting for a refill that happens through a period of rest; usually through prolonged sleep.

If we look at energy as money then the "currency" of energy in the body comes in the form of the chemical called Adenosine Tri-Phosphate or ATP (3 Phosphate molecules). Now imagine using a pound coin to buy a bar of chocolate. As the pound breaks down to its change, you get your chocolate (energy). Similarly, the pound coin in the body is ATP.

All living organisms carry ATP. Energy is created by a cell when ATP is broken down to ADP, which is Adenosine Di-phosphate. This is produced when an ATP breaks down one of its three phosphate molecules when a cell requires energy to perform a function. (think of the pound coin breaking down into change to buy the chocolate).

Now that the phosphate molecule's energy has been released, it can be used on behalf of the cell. When a cell has excess energy, it stores it by attaching a free phosphate molecule to ADP and converting it back into ATP.

The use of energy around the body will vary from task to task and organ to organ. The Basal Metabolic Rate (BMR) measures the total daily energy expenditure per day by the body in a rested state. So basically this is the amount of energy needed just to stay alive and maintain vital functions such as breathing, thinking, heart beating, etc., in other words, minimum functions.

So a minimum amount of energy is needed by the body. With stress activities and energy expenditure the metabolic rate rises, but the BMR remains the same. This means that you have to have a certain amount of energy just to function and any surplus is extra. Once this "extra" energy is gone then you are fatigued and need a recharge. Your body is not going to dip into the energy needed for vital functioning such as breathing or filtering by the kidneys.

So the real question here is "What is depleting my energy?"

Fatigue can be broadly classified into 3 main areas, Physical, Mental and Psychological.

Here are a list of triggers to think about and some quick-fix ideas. Remember these ideas are just pointers, a framework if you like for you to think and research and eventually action as you move forward.

Everyone is different and fatigue affects people in different ways.

Physical Fatigue:

Lack of Sleep: Aim for 7-9 hours of quality sleep each night. Maintain a consistent sleep schedule, create a relaxing bedtime routine, and avoid stimulating activities or electronic devices before bedtime. See the Sleep Hygiene section talked about in the Hot Flushes and Night Sweats section.

Sedentary Lifestyle: Incorporate regular physical activity into your daily routine, such as walking, cycling, or yoga, to boost energy levels and reduce physical fatigue. Activity will naturally tire you out and promote a good night's sleep, which will make you feel more refreshed and generally more capable of handling the day.

Lack of Physical Activity or Excessive Physical Activity: Engage in light to moderate exercise regularly but no more as this in itself will be a trigger for fatigue and exhaustion. Physical activity can improve cardiovascular health, muscle strength, and overall energy levels.

Fluids: Stay adequately hydrated by drinking water throughout the day. Avoid excessive consumption of caffeinated beverages, which can make you urinate, or sugary beverages which affect your insulin and cortisol levels which ultimately leads to fatigue. Limit alcohol intake and avoid drinking close to bedtime to improve sleep quality and prevent fatigue.

Poor Nutrition: Eat a balanced diet with a variety of nutrient-dense foods, including fruits, vegetables, whole grains, lean proteins, and healthy fats. Whilst this is common knowledge, perhaps ask yourself how much are you following the advice. It is balanced because you are getting all the macro-nutrients and micro-nutrients your body needs to work optimally and to help stay resilient. If you are unsure of your current nutritional status, a dietitian or nutritionist will help steer you on the correct path to nutritional wellness.

Skipping Meals: Eat regular, well-balanced meals, without excessive poor carbs to maintain stable blood sugar levels and prevent energy crashes.

Vitamin and mineral deficiency: This includes iron, magnesium zinc all the B vitamins, and vitamin D. This is not exhaustive but a start. A blood test will reveal any deficiencies as well as any hormone issues such as an underactive thyroid.

Obesity: Moving and carrying a large bodily mass takes effort and energy. Adopt a healthy eating plan and engage in regular physical activity to manage weight and increase overall energy levels. As your weight falls there will be a corresponding rise in energy levels as your motivation increases and general sluggishness diminishes.

Chemical Abuse: Smoking, Drinking, and Drugs including Caffeine: Seek support and resources to quit any form of drug abuse, as these habits can negatively affect your body beyond just energy levels. Look at government guidelines determine your safe limits and see if you go beyond this.

Poor Gut Health: You hear a lot about macros but not enough is talked about micro-nutrients. Focus on a diet that is wide and rich in fibre and probiotics to support gut health, as an unhealthy gut can affect overall well-being and energy levels. Adding complex slow-releasing carbohydrates such as beans, sweet potatoes, etc. provides a sustained release of energy rather than spikes in blood sugar from quick-releasing carbs such as breakfast cereals, sugar-loaded foods, and cheap takeaways. A healthy gut means healthy microbiome levels. The gut bacteria are crucial to keeping up levels of the happy hormones serotonin and melatonin needed for sleep.

Excessive Consumption of Heavy Meals: Opt for lighter, balanced meals to prevent post-meal fatigue and promote digestion. It takes a lot of energy to digest a heavy meal. Heavy carb-loaded meals will promote lethargy and sluggishness.

Anything in excess: We are designed to be in balance with our environment, too much of anything puts us in imbalance. For example how many people who have overslept complain of feeling tired or exhausted? How many people who overeat feel sick? How many people who overdo it at the gym are left exhausted and sore? The list goes on. Knowing your limits will at least keep you in a boundary that you are aware of and that you can manage and control.

Medical Conditions and Medications: There are many medical conditions, too numerous to list here that will contribute to fatigue. Chat with your doctor or pharmacist regarding your issues including medications. Do some digging as this can be a big drain on your internal battery. Common medical conditions may include diabetes mellitus, thyroid disorders, autoimmune conditions, adrenal fatigue (not classified as a condition), anaemia, fibromyalgia, obesity, and respiratory disease.

Mental Fatigue:

A combination of Physical and Mental Fatigue leads to "Burnout".

Chronic Stress: practise stress management techniques such as meditation, deep breathing, mindfulness, or yoga to reduce stress and mental fatigue. Keep the battery full by doing less than you need to and finding inner calm.

Anxiety and Depression. Practices like mindfulness, CBT, and better gut health through proper eating all contribute towards helping reduce anxiety and depression in a better way than with medications.

Emotional Exhaustion: Prioritise self-care, and set boundaries! Engage in activities that bring joy and relaxation to combat emotional fatigue.

Overworking or Long Work Hours: Establish a healthy work-life balance, take breaks during work hours, and avoid excessive overtime to prevent mental fatigue. Speak to your boss and change your schedule!

Irregular Sleep Schedule: Maintain a consistent sleep routine, even on weekends, to regulate circadian rhythms and improve mental alertness.

Visual/Excessive Screen Time: Limit screen time, especially before bedtime, to improve sleep quality and reduce mental fatigue.

Excessive Use of Stimulants or Energy Drinks: Limit caffeine and stimulant intake, as excessive use can lead to energy crashes and mental exhaustion. Limit caffeine intake to no more than two cups before midday and alcohol on the weekends or only with meals following government guidelines on intake.

Psychological Fatigue:

Lack of Relaxation and Leisure Time: Prioritise relaxation activities such as hobbies, meditation, or spending time in nature to reduce psychological fatigue. Psychological connections are important not just for energy maintenance but also to stave off loneliness and dementia.

Unhealthy Relationships Set boundaries and seek support to address unhealthy relationships, as they can contribute to psychological fatigue. Ask the hard questions to yourself as only you can fix the issues.

Disrupted Circadian Rhythms: A Circadian rhythm is the internal clock our brains keep to regulate cycles of sleepiness and alertness. This is through responding to changes in daylight in our environment. Maintain a regular sleep schedule and practise good sleep hygiene to regulate circadian rhythms and improve psychological well-being.

Excessive Noise or Light Pollution: Create a calm and soothing environment by reducing noise and light disturbances during sleep and relaxation times.

Excessive Use of Electronic Devices before Bedtime: Limit screen time before bedtime to promote better sleep quality and psychological well-being. Sleeping is meant to be just that, not watching TV in bed or checking e-mails.

As this list is not exhaustive, you may need to add some of your own to categorise.

We now need to isolate where the fatigue is coming from and the times of day it is arising.

Because fatigue can be a side effect of another menopausal issue such as say poor sleep, then once that other issue is dealt with the fatigue may automatically start improving or even resolving itself.

Again we are adopting the same strategies as before:

The Action Plan is:

Start Using Tools from Day 1
Change Trigger factors you can Control
Monitor progression and the end of each week

Roadmap

Reflection and starting weekend before Week 1 Saturday Day 1 Sunday Day 2	• Decide your goal for Fatigue Reduction • Start morning tool (am) • Fill in the Fatigue Disruption Sheet • Am + Pm tools • Start reviewing Fatigue Triggers including your regular diet
Week 1-4 (6) Monday-Friday	• Am and Pm tools daily • Daily fatigue tracking and changing of triggers
Saturday and Sunday of each week	• Every weekend review the Fatigue Diary and check your progress making the changes for the following week
WEEK 4 or 6	• Review progress by going back to the Initial Fatigue Disruption Sheet you completed on Day 1

My Goal is ....

Start by monitoring using the following Fatigue Disruption Monitoring Sheet: This is a before and after rating to see where you are before and after doing this course.

Think back last week and answer the following:

How bad is my fatigue on a scale of 0 to 10, with 0 being none and 10 being severe.

0	1	2	3	4	5	6	7	8	9	10
none/mild					moderate			severe/unbearable		

How much of a disruption does it make on your life a scale of 0-10

0	1	2	3	4	5	6	7	8	9	10
none/mild					moderate			severe/unbearable		

Important! List some of your exact thoughts by the words you use (this is important as you will see later),your feelings and behaviours around these events (as many as you like) and then score them in terms of severity and disruption.

If you have already used CBT for hot flushes then you know about changing of the thoughts.

Situation	Exact Thought Wording	Feelings	Behaviour	Severity 0-10	Disruption 0-10
feel wiped out	why me? what have I done to deserve this?	despair	struggling to get out of bed	8	9

Table 13: Fatigue Disruption Monitoring

We now need to isolate where the fatigue is coming from and the times of day it is arising. Over the next 4-6 weeks start tracking your daily habits to see when and where the fatigue arises.

Here is a suggested diary:

Menopausal Fatigue Diary

Date	Description of Issue	Notes
Sleep Quality and Hours of Sleep	Rate your sleep quality last night From 1-10	
Hot Flushes/Night Sweats	Rate the severity of hot flashes or night sweats experienced today (1 (mild) - 10 (severe))	
Energy Levels	Rate your energy levels throughout the day (1 (low) - 10 (high))	
-Morning		
-Afternoon		
-Evening		
Stress and Mood	Rate your overall stress and mood today (1 (low) - 10 (high))	
Physical Activity	Make a list of physical activities done today and how they have made you feel	
Diet	List your meals and snacks today and how they have made you feel	
Menopausal Symptoms	List any menopausal symptoms you experienced today (e.g., mood swings, vaginal dryness, etc.) and how you felt	
Medications/Supplements	List any medications or supplements you took today and their dosage and how they made you feel	
What type of Fatigue felt (physical, mental, psychological)		

Table 14: Menopausal Fatigue Diary

At the end of each week start asking the hard questions. Remember to ask "If not, why not?" after each question; here are a few examples:

What triggers have I actively reduced this week?

....

....

....

Did I work out what type of fatigue I may be suffering from?

....

....

....

Did I give myself enough breaks during work?

....

....

....

Did I stick to my goal today of e.g., no coffee or light exercise?

....

....

....

Did I speak to my boss about rearranging my work schedule or dropping some hours?

....

....

....

How do I feel? Do I need to seek help?

....

....

....

Did I make time self care for example a massage?

....

....

....

How much of a discomfort am I putting up with before taking action?

....

....

....

Am I giving myself enough sleep?

....

....

....

There are a myriad of questions you could be asking yourself. By taking a long hard look, trying to change triggers, and using the tools you should be able to improve your quality of life around your fatigue. As long as you are moving forward and taking action you are progressing.

Weeks 4-6 Review

So by now with diligent action you should have made progress compared to where you started from. Now is the time to revisit the initial Fatigue Disruption Monitoring Sheet again, the one you filled in on Day 1.

How bad is my fatigue on a scale of 0 to 10, with 0 being none and 10 being severe.

0   1   2   3   4   5   6   7   8   9   10
none/mild   moderate   severe/unbearable

How much of a disruption does it make on your life a scale of 0-10

0   1   2   3   4   5   6   7   8   9   10
none/mild   moderate   severe/unbearable

Now review the exact thought wordings you use daily. How have they changed from the initial sheet?

Situation	Exact Thought Wording	Feelings	Behaviour	Severity 0-10	Disruption 0-10
can't stop yawning	why me? what have I done to deserve this?	despair	struggling to get out of bed	8	9

Table 15: Fatigue Disruption Monitoring Revisited

In cases of chronic and unexplained fatigue, it's essential to consult a healthcare professional for a thorough evaluation to determine the underlying cause and develop a comprehensive treatment plan.

This now concludes module around reducing menopausal fatigue.

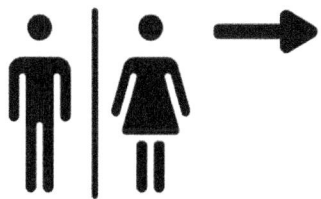

GENITO-URINARY ISSUES

Tools to be used

Kegel Exercises
Bladder Training and Monitoring
Review Diet, Triggers and Eating Patterns

It is important to note that the action plan is only a beginners guide to pelvic health. Relief that is not obtained from the information given below should be an indication that you need to seek professional help in this area. Remember you **must** inform your doctor of any bleeding in this area, please do not ignore this.

In the main section of the book, I covered incontinence and it's various types. Before we move onto strengthening the pelvic floor area to help reduce an overactive bladder, there are a few other issues I would like to touch upon.

Modification of Diet

Your diet can play a crucial role in your pelvic health. If you do not incorporate enough fibre and fluid in your daily eating patterns then you are at risk of constipation. This will lead to straining when you go to the loo and this puts direct pressure on the pelvic floor area. An intake of at least 25-30g of fibre and at least 1.5 l of water daily, is a minimum requirement to keep your bowels moving in a healthy direction. You can buy fibre supplements if you cannot meet the daily intake requirements through fruit and vegetables.

Also, consider pumpkin seeds; their oil has phytochemicals that appear to reduce bladder muscle contractions and inflammation. To help reduce urinary infections consider foods such as cranberry and vitamin C which help acidify the urine and ward off infections. There is research to support that certain beverages such as tea, coffee, soda (including diet), and alcohol help to irritate the lining of the bladder and in general should be avoided where possible. (Cardozo L. 2011)

Controlling Urination for Urge Incontinence

A way to help retrain your bladder is just by holding on when you get the urge to pee. This will allow over time for your bladder to hold onto more urine as you progressively ignore the signals to go. Please check with your doctor that you are clinically fit to try this and it is appropriate to do so.

Start by knowing approximately how much you are going to urinate over a length of time. So for example a visual representation of 500ml of water would be a bottle of coke. Now drink this on an empty stomach and wait to see when you urinate and approximately how much.

Your bladder can hold roughly 400-450ml of fluid before it needs to be emptied. You may need to pee in a container the first time around to get an idea of volume. After you've done this a few times, you'll know how much you'll need to urinate based on the volume you drank. You can save yourself for times when you've had a lot to drink and need to go by ignoring, say, small amounts of volume.

Practise holding and delaying in a few-minute increments. But also be aware that it is perfectly normal and necessary to go to the bathroom. This is about your ability to exert self-control over the urges.

Remember to keep liners on the ready until you have more of a rhythm and know your urges. Your doctor can also help by providing medication and other alternatives if you need it. Also, bladder infections are going to be more common in the menopausal phase so be aware that this is a potential trigger point for incontinence as well.

Vaginal Dryness

We have already explored some of the reasons for vaginal dryness, so how can we help to provide relief in the area? There are two pathways a woman could potentially go on, either the hormonal route to replace the oestrogen loss or non-hormonal treatment which are currently on the market. In my experience, I would recommend both with a bit of experimenting. Start with non-hormonal treatments first and then the hormonal.

The normal HRT route is where you either take tablets from your doctor and expect the symptoms to settle down after a few months or there is the localised application of Oestrogen.

If we are looking just to alleviate genito-urinary symptoms then the localised application in the vaginal area is a lower-risk option compared to normal HRT tablets. Compared to the oral route, there is less absorption into the body from this area which means reducing your risk of clots and potentially cancer.

A daily application of the hormone can then be reduced with the introduction of a non-hormonal-based product so in effect, reducing your risk even further. Localised oestrogen is available as pessaries, vaginal creams, gels, or vaginal tablets.

Experiment initially with the dose of hormone that settles your symptoms and then slowly withdraw daily but at the same time add the non-hormonal treatment until you find that balance between symptom resolution and hormonal usage. This may take a little time of experimenting but will be worth it long term.

Here is a **list of non-hormonal treatments** available in the UK to treat vaginal dryness:

Vaginal Moisturisers: These are designed to maintain vaginal moisture and can be used regularly, regardless of age and sexual activity. They help to keep the tissues well-hydrated and feeling less sore. Examples include Replens and Sliquid. (Hormone Health 2023, NHS Choices 2021)

Vaginal Lubricants: These are specifically designed to reduce friction during sexual intercourse and can be used as needed. They are different from moisturisers as they are not intended for regular use to maintain vaginal moisture. Examples include K-Y Liquibeads. (Hazell 2023)

Ospemifene (Osphena): This is a non-hormonal oral medication that has been shown to relieve symptoms of moderate to severe vaginal atrophy. In the United States and at the time of writing, It is the first and only FDA-approved, once-daily, oral, non-hormonal treatment to treat both moderate to severe vaginal dryness and/or painful intercourse due to menopause. (Duchesnay USA 2023)

Dehydroepiandrosterone (DHEA): This is used daily as a vaginal pessary and works instead of oestrogen. It is a precursor to testosterone.

Laser Treatment: This is called "Fractional CO2" laser treatment. It has been suggested it can redevelop the vaginal tissue, increase collagen production, and bring the vagina back to its normal functioning. This is anything but cheap but is available as an option.

When looking for a lubricant, I generally say to women who ask for my recommendations to treat the vaginal area as if you are buying a cream to treat the skin on your arm which is also dry and sore.

On your arm, use a very small amount of product and test a very small area. Now wait and see how your skin reacts, you should know within half an hour or so whether the product agrees with you.

In the same manner, use a very small amount of vaginal lubricant in a readily accessible part of the vagina. This is in case you have to quickly remove it and wash it off; the last thing you want is a product that will sting or burn and make the area worse.

Once you have found a suitable product, use it frequently and be generous with the amount, especially before intercourse. Choose a ph balanced product with the least amount of ingredients, so no perfumes or additives, nothing that may "arouse or waken" the sexual experience, so nothing flavoured or tingly.

Just remember you may need to try and heal as well as nourish the area first before attempting the sexual experience.

Be aware of the following though: Glycerine may cause yeast infections, Nonoxynol-9 may irritate and cause inflammation, and Vaseline/Baby oil is a no-no as well as these may damage condoms. Parabens and Chlorhexidine have been suggested as red flags due to irritation and parabens being a cancer risk. (Citations E)

Check for reviews and experiment a little to find the one that suits you.

Vaginal Pain

Alexey Welsh has worked for over 20 years as a holistic sex coach and an alternative sex therapist. He describes in his YouTube video the 5 different patterns of vaginal pain experienced by a woman of any age. This may be particularly relevant in the menopause.

1. Friction Pain: this is a result of chaffing of the vagina from the penis due to insufficient lubrication. This may be due to the vagina itself being too dry or not using enough of an external lubricating agent. He emphasises that the woman needs to be properly aroused for this to happen or to maintain enough external lubrication right from the start and during the entire sexual experience.

2. Tightness Pain: this is where the entrance to the vagina is tight and the penis is comparatively large to the area being entered.

This stretches the vagina uncomfortably leading to pain. Women who suffer this may not have had sex in a while, or they may just have a narrower vagina, or it may just be that the penis is larger than the vagina can comfortably accommodate.

Either way, it can lead to pain and even micro-tearing in the area. This type of pain is immediate on penetration even with lubrication. Men will feel like an elastic band has been tied around their penis. To relieve this, he recommends starting carefully and "pace", in other words gentle sex to expand the area in question. However, the best method appears to be penetration without a full erection. Now this may be a little challenging for men as the whole point of a full erection is for penetration. So a semi-hard penis may be the way to go with lubrication here. Vaginal elasticity will improve with the frequency of sex.

3. Vaginismus: not to be confused with tightness, this type of pain is brought about by the body's fear of penetration. The vaginal muscles will tighten up automatically when any type of penetration is attempted for example a tampon. Vaginismus is a contraction of the vagina rather than the vagina being tight or small in size in the first place and is mainly due to anxiety, trauma, or intimacy issues and based around your feelings of penetration. This is a tricky and complex area and may need specialised help to alleviate the anxiety. Vaginal dilators may not be enough as simply thinking about fearing penetration may set up the contraction. Relaxation techniques at the moment will also be helpful.

4. Cervical Pain: Alexey describes this as "crashing" into the wall at the back of the vagina, and the feeling of being bruised there. There could be both physical and emotional trauma that may have been set up through previous encounters. Relief can be

partially emotional but also by reducing the depth of penetration from the male partner. The male partner should experiment with movement, sexual positions, and penetration depth until the woman feels comfortable, which may also help relieve the emotional aspect of this type of pain. Communication is key for both parties.

5. Burning Pain: this appears to be most trickiest to solve. It can be located anywhere in the vagina and appears even with lubrication and careful gentle sex. Alexey suggests this is due to a hypersensitivity of the nerves in the areas of pain. This is opposed to Vulvodynia where this is happening in the area of the vulva only. Burning pain can be experienced anywhere in the vaginal area. This is due to a disorder of the nervous system and there are several options here from medications to local anaesthetic creams or gels and is best discussed with a health professional like your doctor or a sex therapist.

You can see the actual video on YouTube at.... https://youtu.be/94nWwmrqD0k?feature=shared

Alexey has many other videos around sexual health on his channel Alexey Welsh, please go and check him out.

Bladder Leakage Triggers

As before, let's take a look at what can trigger bladder leakage and what you can change immediately

Some common triggers taken from Healthline.com and the Mayo Clinic include:

1. Caffeine: Consuming beverages like coffee, tea, and energy drinks that contain caffeine can irritate the bladder and increase the frequency of urination, potentially leading to leakage.

2. Alcohol: Alcohol is a diuretic that increases urine production and can irritate the bladder, causing urgency and leakage.

3. Spicy and acidic foods: Spicy foods, citrus fruits, tomatoes, and carbonated drinks can irritate the bladder and worsen incontinence symptoms.

4. Medications: Certain medications, such as diuretics, sedatives, muscle relaxants, and blood pressure medications, can affect bladder control and contribute to leakage.

5. High-impact exercises: Activities like running, jumping, and high-intensity workouts can put pressure on the bladder and lead to stress incontinence.

6. Chronic coughing: Conditions like chronic bronchitis, asthma, or smoking can cause frequent bouts of coughing, which can put pressure on the bladder and result in leakage.

7. Obesity: Being overweight can increase the pressure on the bladder and weaken the pelvic floor muscles, leading to stress incontinence.

According to research, a 3-5% weight loss reduction can decrease urinary incontinence episodes by about 50% (Aoki et al. 2017).

Menopausal changes: Hormonal fluctuations during menopause can contribute to urinary incontinence in women.

Please note that it is important to consult with a healthcare professional for an accurate diagnosis and personalised advice regarding bladder leakage triggers and management.

The Action Plan is:

Start Using Tools from Day 1
Change Trigger factors you can Control
Monitor progression and the end of each week

Roadmap

Reflection and starting weekend before Week 1 Saturday Day 1 Sunday Day 2	• Decide your goal for your GU issues • Start Kegels (am) • Fill in Disruption Sheet • Kegels in Am + Pm • Bladder training throughout the day • Review Bladder Triggers including your regular diet
Week 1-4 (6) Monday-Friday	• Kegels am and pm daily • Bladder training throughout the day • Daily monitoring and changing of triggers
Saturday and Sunday of each week	• Every weekend complete the Adjustment Diary and review your progress making the changes for the following week
WEEK 4 or 6	• Review progress by going back to the Initial Sheet you filled on Day 1

VERY IMPORTANT! **Please do not perform Kegel exercises if you suffer any kind of pain, during urination, with an overactive pelvic floor, or any pelvic floor dysfunction.** If you are not sure please seek advice. As before let's grade the issue by filling in the Bladder Disruption Sheet:

This is a before and after rating to see where you are before and after doing this course.

Think back last week and answer the following:

How bad is my incontinence on a scale of 0 to 10, with 0 being none and 10 being severe.

0   1   2   3   4   5   6   7   8   9   10
none/mild   moderate   severe/unbearable

How much of a disruption does it make on your life a scale of 0-10

0   1   2   3   4   5   6   7   8   9   10
none/mild   moderate   severe/unbearable

Important! List some of your exact thoughts by the words you use (this is important as you will see later),your feelings and behaviours around these events (as many as you like) and then score them in terms of severity and disruption.

If you have already used CBT for hot flushes then you know about changing of the thoughts.

Situation	Exact Thought Wording	Feelings	Behaviour	Severity 0-10	Disruption 0-10
leakage at work	oh god! not again	helplessness	change clothing	7	10

Table 16: Genito-Urinary Disruption Monitoring

Urinary Symptoms Diary

Here is a suggested diary you can use to track whether your exercises are working for you. You may need some extra help from your doctor if you find the exercises are not enough.

Remember to review your triggers and make the necessary changes and do the exercises at the same time to maximise your results.

Use the grading to monitor your desire to want to go to the loo.

Desire to void
1= I need to go now!
2= I can wait 10 minutes
3= I can wait up to 20 minutes

Volume of Urine Output
1= small amount e.g., drops
2= medium amount e.g., underwear/protection damp
3= large amount e.g., underwear/protection soaked

this grading is in the diary below

Daily Diary

Day and Date...........

Time of the Day	What I drank e.g., Tea	Volume Drank approximately in ml	Urge to go Grading 1 2 3	Volume of Urine approximately 1 2 3	What tools did I use e.g., Kegels exercise	Any Medication Used	Any other causative factors e.g., exercise	Any Notes e.g., what's working/not
6-7 am								
7-8 am								
8-9 am								
9-10 am								
10-11 am								
11-12 am								
12-1 pm								
1-2 pm								
2-3 pm								

3-4 pm								
4-5 pm								
5-6 pm								
6-7 pm								
7-8 pm								
8-9 pm								
9-10 pm								
10-11 pm								
11-12 pm								
12-1 am								
1-2 am								
2-3 am								
3-4 am								
4-5 am								
5-6 am								

Table 17: Urinary Symptom Diary

Weeks 4-6 Review

Hopefully by now you should have made progress compared to where you started from. Now is the time to revisit the initial Bladder Disruption Sheet again, the one you filled in on Day 1.

How bad is my Incontinence now on a scale of 0 to 10, with 0 being none and 10 being severe.

0	1	2	3	4	5	6	7	8	9	10
none/mild					moderate			severe/unbearable		

How much of a disruption does it make on your life a scale of 0-10

0	1	2	3	4	5	6	7	8	9	10
none/mild					moderate			severe/unbearable		

Now review the exact thought wordings you use daily. How have they changed from the initial sheet?

Situation	Exact Thought Wording	Feelings	Behaviour	Severity 0-10	Disruption 0-10
leakage at work	oh god! not again	helplessness	change clothing	7	10

Table 18: Genito-Urinary Disruption Monitoring Revisited

This is a process and will take time and practise. Use the power of your mindset to propel you forward.

The beauty around bladder and pelvic floor training is that this can be done all day every day, and very discreetly.

Go easy on yourself, the pelvic floor area has reduced it's tone for whatever reason and getting that back to a former time will take training, just like going to the gym but without the gym drama. Don't punish yourself if you are not achieving results straight away.

This now concludes the treatment module around reducing genito-urinary issues.

We have now finished the Action component of the book.

So as we bring to an end this action-packed journey through holistic practices and behavioural changes, take a moment to appreciate the strides you've made.

I congratulate you if you have made it this far.

Over these past 4-6 weeks, you've not only embraced change but actively cultivated a holistic approach to navigating the areas we have covered.

I hope you have found the information useful and informative. Remember that these practices aren't just temporary fixes; they're enduring tools in your arsenal, empowering you to carry on navigating your issues whenever you need to.

Remember to seek out further help including support, supplements, and medications where necessary.

Thank you for your participation, I hope this has made a significant impact on your menopausal journey.

To find out more information about me and of how I am trying to help women over 45 with their health and weight, please visit **www.sisstas.com.**

EPILOGUE

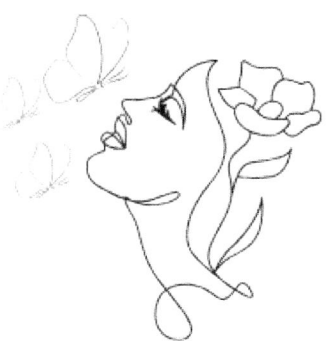

I know that many women look upon menopause with trepidation and dread. From those I have had the privilege of talking to, they also had to live with the confusion, inadequate support from both medical and allied health professions, and always the spectre of health risks that HRT brings along with it.

I hope this book will give you some inspiration that alternative practices can and will make a real difference to your menopausal life, at whatever stage you are in.

Look upon this journey as a one of self-discovery and move forward with a sense of purpose and accomplishment. By taking the necessary and well-deserved time for self-care, I am confident that you will achieve many of the goals outlined in this book.

The menopause will bring its daily challenges. There are a multitude of stories of women venting their issues. While these symptoms may cause varying levels of disruption, I hope you can see that they are signalling a change in this now, second chapter of your life.

With our cash-strapped NHS, and time-poor health professionals, take the reins yourself and feel empowered to take action. Please don't wait for someone else to come and fix these issues, do it for yourself! As the L'oreal advert keeps telling us all "You're worth it".

You will be faced with challenges that the ageing process brings so the earlier you start the better your outcome will be in the long term. This is an investment for your future self.

There is far too much hate and shaming in the media. Remember to go easy on yourself, the human body is an incredibly complex machine and everything takes time. This is a journey every woman will go on and every woman will feel the change in herself. It is not some sort of self-inflicted curse or punishment nor should it be viewed that way.

I know you will embrace this new way of life and forge ahead to meet these challenges, which go beyond the HRT drum that is constantly beating around us.

Life is an adventure, and you're the protagonist of your story.

I wish you the very best of luck moving forward!

A SMALL FAVOUR FOR AMAZON PURCHASERS

"Dear Reader, if you've enjoyed this book, I'd be immensely grateful if you could spare a moment (literally 5 seconds) to share your thoughts with others on Amazon.
Reviews from wonderful customers like you can make a huge difference and help empower other readers in their menopausal journey. Thank you deeply for your kind words, time and support!"

If you have an Amazon account and you have spent $50, then it is very simple:

For Paperback/Hardback

1. Open up the camera setting on your phone and look for the scanner icon.
2. Scan the QR code below appropriate to the country where you purchased the book.
3. Leave a review, and that's it, simple!

For Amazon UK

For Amazon USA

For Amazon Canada

For Amazon Australia

For Amazon Germany

For Amazon France

For Amazon India

For Amazon Mexico

For Amazon UAE

For Amazon
Saudi Arabia

For Amazon Japan

Thank You!

RESOURCES

W herever you are in your menopausal journey, there maybe times where you need extra support. Here are some resources to be aware of. You may find more local organisations depending upon where in the world you are reading this book from and the type of support you need.

International Menopause Society
Rebecca Cheshire, IMS CEO
13 Leechwell Street, Totnes, Devon TQ9 5SX, UK
E-mail: email@imsociety.org

The British Menopause Society
The Barn, Dukes Place, Marlow, UK
https://thebms.org.uk/
Phone 01628 890199

European Menopause and Andropause Society
c/o K.I.T. Group GmbH
Association & Conference Management
Kurfürstendamm 71
10709 Berlin, Germany

+49 30 246 03-0
+49 30 246 03-200
emas@kit-group.org

The North American Menopause Society
30050 Chagrin Blvd., Suite 120W
Pepper Pike, OH 44124, USA
Phone: 440/442-7550
Fax: 440/442-2660
Email: info@menopause.org

Canadian Menopause Society / Société Canadienne de Ménopause
Mailing Address: #171-1089 West Broadway, Vancouver BC V6H 1E5
Temporary office address: Carey Centre on UBC Campus, Unit 218 - 5920 Iona Drive, Vancouver, BC. V6T 1J6
Phone: 604-818-1834
Email: info@sigmamenopause.com

Australasian Menopause Society (for Australia and New Zealand)
Phone: 61 3 5962 6241
Post: PO Box 280, Healesville VIC 3777
Email: Australasian Menopause Society: ams@menopause.org.au

Indian Menopause Society
C/O Paresh Patel,
Office Assistant, IMS,
D-302, Uma Residency, Near Mark Point,
Karadwa Gam Road,
Dindoli, Surat - 394210
Contact 9949621094

South African Menopause Society
SAMS Secretariat: ROYAL HOUSE
P O Box 1927, Country Club, Durban, SA 4302
Phone: 082 553 8201
Email: info@menopause.co.za

The Menopause Charity
Adamson House
Towers Business Park
Wilmslow Road
Manchester M20 2YY, UK.
https://www.themenopausecharity.org/

The Daisy Network
PO BOX 71432,
London SW6 9HJ
https://www.daisynetwork.org/

Worldwide Cancer Research
1st Floor, Canning Exchange
10 Canning Street
Edinburgh EH3 8EG
https://www.worldwidecancerresearch.org/

https://www.nhs.uk/

Royal Osteoporosis Society
St. James House, Lower Bristol Road,
Bath BA2 3BH. UK
https://theros.org.uk/

Relate National (for Mental Health)
76 St Giles Street,
Northampton,
NN1 1JW, UK
https://www.relate.org.uk/

Hub Of Hope (mental health support database for the UK)
https://hubofhope.co.uk/

British Thyroid Foundation
Suite 12, One Sceptre House
Hornbeam Square North
Hornbeam Park
Harrogate
HG2 8PB
https://www.btf-thyroid.org/

British Heart Foundation
Compton House
2300 The Crescent
Birmingham Business Park
Birmingham
B37 7YE
https://www.bhf.org.uk/

World Health Organisation (WHO) Headquarters in Geneva
Avenue Appia 20
1211 Geneva
Switzerland
Telephone: +41 22 791 21 11
https://www.who.int/

UK Council for Psychotherapy
2 America Square
London
EC3N 2LU
https://www.psychotherapy.org.uk/

REFERENCES

Amabebe E, Anumba DOC. The Vaginal Microenvironment: The Physiologic Role of Lactobacilli. Front Med (Lausanne). 2018 Jun 13;5:181. doi: 10.3389/fmed.2018.00181. PMID: 29951482; PMCID: PMC6008313.

American College of Obstetricians and Gynaecologists. (2020). Practice Bulletin No. 155: Urinary Incontinence in Women. Obstetrics & Gynecology, 135(5), e155–e168. DOI: 10.1097/AOG.0000000000003838

Aoki Y, Brown HW, Brubaker L, Cornu JN, Daly JO, Cartwright R. Urinary incontinence in women. Nat Rev Dis Primers. 2017 Nov 16;3:17097

Aron A, Norman CC, Aron EN, McKenna C, Heyman RE. Couples' shared participation in novel and arousing activities and experienced relationship quality. J Pers Soc Psychol. 2000 Feb;78(2):273-84. doi: 10.1037//0022-3514.78.2.273. PMID: 10707334.

Bailey, Ryan. "Testosterone: 15 Best Foods to Eat for Better T-Levels - Men's Health." Menshealth.Com/Uk, 2023,

www.menshealth.com/uk/nutrition/a747704/boost-
testosterone-foods/.

Bansal R, Aggarwal N. Menopausal Hot Flashes: A Concise
Review. J Midlife Health. 2019 Jan-Mar;10(1):6-13. doi:
10.4103/jmh.JMH_7_19. PMID: 31001050; PMCID:
PMC6459071.

Bea, J.W. et al. 2011, Effect of hormone therapy on lean body
mass, falls, and fractures: Six-year results from the Women's
Health Initiative Hormone Trials. Menopause, 18(1), pp. 44-52.

Benedetti MG, Furlini G, Zati A, Letizia Mauro G. The
Effectiveness of Physical Exercise on Bone Density in
Osteoporotic Patients. Biomed Res Int. 2018 Dec
23;2018:4840531. doi: 10.1155/2018/4840531. PMID: 30671455;
PMCID: PMC6323511.

Breast Cancer. Org. "Using HRT (Hormone Replacement
Therapy) ." Breast Cancer Risk and Hormone Replacement
Therapy: What You Need to Know, 2023,
www.breastcancer.org/risk/risk-factors/using-hormone-
replacement-therapy.

Brzezinski A, Adlercreutz H, Shaoul R, et al. Short-term effects
of phytoestrogen-rich diet on postmenopausal women.
Menopause. 1997;4(2):89–94.

Burger, H. G. (1999). The endocrinology of the menopause.
Maturitas, 34, S115-S120.

Burke LE, Wang J, Sevick MA. Self-monitoring in weight loss: a
systematic review of the literature. J Am Diet Assoc. 2011
Jan;111(1):92-102. doi: 10.1016/j.jada.2010.10.008. PMID:
21185970; PMCID: PMC3268700.

Burns, D. D. (1980). Feeling good: The new mood therapy. New York, NY: New American Library.

C.J. Haines, L. Rong, T.K.H. Chung, D.H.Y. Leung,

C.J.H. Martin et al. (eds.), Nutrition and Diet in Menopause, Nutrition and Health, 101 DOI 10.1007/978-1-62703-373-2_8, © Springer Science+Business Media New York 2013

Cacioppo JT, Cacioppo S, Gollan JK. The negativity bias: Conceptualization, quantification, and individual differences. Behavioural and Brain Sciences. 2014;37(3):309-310. doi:10.1017/s0140525x13002537

Cancer Research UK. "Hormones and Cancer." Cancer Research UK, 2023, www.cancerresearchuk.org/about-cancer/causes-of-cancer/hormones-and-cancer/does-hormone-replacement-therapy-increase-cancer-risk.

Cannon, W. B. (1929). Organization for physiological homeostasis. Physiological Reviews, 9(3), 399-431.

Cardozo L. Systematic review of overactive bladder therapy in females. Can Urol Assoc J. 2011 Oct;5(5 Suppl 2):S139-42. doi: 10.5489/cuaj.11185. PMID: 21989527; PMCID: PMC3193389.

Chopra S, Sharma KA, Ranjan P, Malhotra A, Vikram NK, Kumari A. Weight Management Module for Perimenopausal Women: A Practical Guide for Gynecologists. J Midlife Health. 2019 Oct-Dec;10(4):165-172. doi: 10.4103/jmh.JMH_155_19. PMID: 31942151; PMCID: PMC6947726.

Cleary MP, Grossmann ME. Minireview: Obesity and breast cancer: the estrogen connection. Endocrinology. 2009 Jun;150(6):2537-42. doi: 10.1210/en.2009-0070. Epub 2009 Apr 16. PMID: 19372199; PMCID: PMC2689796.

D browska J, D browska-Galas M, Rutkowska M, Michalski BA. Twelve-week exercise training and the quality of life in menopausal women - clinical trial. Prz Menopauzalny. 2016 Mar;15(1):20-5. doi: 10.5114/pm.2016.58769. Epub 2016 Mar 29. PMID: 27095954; PMCID: PMC4828504.

Davinelli S, Nielsen ME, Scapagnini G. Astaxanthin in Skin Health, Repair, and Disease: A Comprehensive Review. Nutrients. 2018 Apr 22;10(4):522. doi: 10.3390/nu10040522. PMID: 29690549; PMCID: PMC5946307.

Dennerstein, L., et al. (2010). A Population-Based Study of Menopausal Symptoms. Obstetrics & Gynecology, 115(2 Pt 1), 249–256. doi: 10.1097/AOG.0b013e3181cbd856.

Drake, M. J., et al. (2017). Physiology and Pathophysiology of the Female Lower Urinary Tract.

Duchesnay USA. "Menopause Symptoms Rubbing You the Wrong Way? Ask Your Healthcare Provider for Osphena®." Osphena, 2033, osphena.com/.

Dumoulin, C., & Hay-Smith, J. (2010). Pelvic floor muscle training versus no treatment, or inactive control treatments, for urinary incontinence in women. Cochrane Database of Systematic Reviews. DOI: 10.1002/14651858.CD005654.pub2

Farage, M. A., & Miller, K. W. (2009). Hormonal therapy for women in menopause. Skin Pharmacology and Physiology, 22(3), 133-146.

Files JA, Ko MG, Pruthi S. Bioidentical hormone therapy. Mayo Clin Proc. 2011 Jul;86(7):673-80, quiz 680. doi: 10.4065/mcp.2010.0714. Epub 2011 Apr 29. PMID: 21531972; PMCID: PMC3127562.

Freedman RR. Behavioural treatment of menopausal hot flushes: evaluation by ambulatory monitoring. Am. J. Obstet. Gynecol. 1992;167:436–439

Freedman, R. R. (2005). Pathophysiology and treatment of menopausal hot flushes. Seminars in Reproductive Medicine, 23(2), 117-125.

Ganceviciene R, Liakou AI, Theodoridis A, Makrantonaki E, Zouboulis CC. Skin anti-ageing strategies. Dermatoendocrinol. 2012 Jul 1;4(3):308-19. doi: 10.4161/derm.22804. PMID: 23467476; PMCID: PMC3583892.

Gartlehner G, Patel SV, Reddy S, Rains C, Schwimmer M, Kahwati L. Hormone Therapy for the Primary Prevention of Chronic Conditions in Postmenopausal Persons: Updated Evidence Report and Systematic Review for the US Preventive Services Task Force. JAMA. 2022;328(17):1747–1765. doi:10.1001/jama.2022.18324tps://www.news-medical.net/?tag=%2FHormone-Replacement-Therapy

Genazzani, A. D., Prati, A., Santagni, S., & Ricchieri, F. (2003). Cholecystokinin-8 tests in postmenopausal women with and without estrogen replacement therapy. Menopause, 10(3), 265-271.

Gold EB, Colvin A, Avis N, Bromberger J, Greendale GA, Powell L, Sternfeld B, Matthews K. Longitudinal analysis of the association between vasomotor symptoms and race/ethnicity across the menopausal transition: study of women's health across the nation. Am. J. Pub. Health. 2006; 96:1–10.

Goldring, M. B., & Otero, M. (2011). Inflammation in osteoarthritis. Current Opinion in Rheumatology, 23(5), 471-478.

Grech A, Sui Z, Rangan A, Simpson SJ, Coogan SCP, Raubenheimer D. Macronutrient imbalance drives energy intake in an obesogenic food environment: An ecological analysis. Obesity (Silver Spring). 2022 Nov;30(11):2156-2166. doi: 10.1002/boy.23578. PMID: 36321270; PMCID: PMC9828743.

Green R, Santoro N. Menopausal Symptoms and Ethnicity: The Study of Women's Health across the Nation. Women's Health. 2009;5(2):127-133. doi:10.2217/17455057.5.2.127

Greendale GA, Huang HM, Wight GR, Zeeman T, Letters C, Avis NE, Johnston J, Llangamarch AS. Effects of the menopause transition and hormone use on cognitive performance in midlife women. Neurology. 2009 May 26;72(21):1850-7. doi: 10.1212/WIL.0b013e3181a71193. PMID: 19470968; PMCID: PMC2690984.

Guyton, A. C., & Hall, J. E. (2006). Textbook of Medical Physiology (11th ed.). Saunders.

Hadjidakis DJ, Androulakis II. Bone remodelling. Ann N Y Cad Sc. 2006 Dec;1092:385-96. doi: 10.1196/annals.1365.035. PMID: 17308163.

Hazell, Dr Toni. "Vaginal Dryness: Symptoms, Causes, and Treatment." Patient. Info, 22 Oct. 2023, patient.info/women-health/menopause/vaginal-dryness-atrophic-vaginitis.

Henderson CW. Cognitive changes after menopause: influence of estrogen. Clin Obstet Gynecol. 2008 Sep;51(3):618-26. doi: 10.1097/GR.0b013e318180ba10. PMID: 18677155; PMCID: PMC2637911.

Henriette van Praag, Exercise and the brain: something to chew on, Trends in Neurosciences, Volume 32, Issue 5, 2009, Pages 283-290, ISSN 0166-2236

Hidalgo-Lopez, E., Mueller, K., Harris, T. et al. Human menstrual cycle variation in subcortical functional brain connectivity: a multimodal analysis approach. Brain Strutt Functor 225, 591–605 (2020). https://dot-org/10.1007/s00429-019-02019-z.

Hodis HM, Mack W. Menopausal Hormone Replacement Therapy and Reduction of All-Cause Mortality and Cardiovascular Disease: It Is About Time and Timing. Cancer J. 2022 May-Jun 01;28(3):208-223. doi: 10.1097/POP.0000000000000591. PMID: 35594469; PMCID: PMC9178928.

Hormone Health. "Vaginal Dryness Treatment: Menopause." Hormone Health, 21 July 2023, hormonehealth.co.uk/dont-suffer-in-silence-what-to-do-about-vaginal-dryness.

Hørslev-Petersen, K. (2008). Rheumatology: A Clinical Handbook. Springer Science & Business Media.

Kołodyńska, G., Zalewski, M., & Rożek-Piechura, K. (2019). Urinary incontinence in postmenopausal women – causes, symptoms, treatment. Menopause Review/Przegląd Menopauzalny, 18(1), 46-50. https://doi.org/10.5114/pm.2019.84157

Kongnyuy et al. (2011). Oestrogen and progestogen hormone replacement therapy for perimenopausal and post-menopausal women: weight and body fat distribution. Cochrane Gynaecology and Fertility Group, 4.

Lauche, R., Langhorst, J., Lee, M. S., Dobos, G., & Cramer, H. (2016). A systematic review and meta-analysis on the effects of yoga on rheumatoid arthritis. Journal of Rheumatology, 43(3), 202-214.

Leonard, Jayne. "The Best Foods to Boost Low Testosterone." Medical News Today, MediLexicon International, 2023, www.medicalnewstoday.com/articles/323759.

Lu CB, Liu PF, Zhou YS, Meng FC, Qiao TY, Yang XJ, Li XY, Xue Q, Xu H, Liu Y, Han Y, Zhang Y. Musculoskeletal Pain during the Menopausal Transition: A Systematic Review and Meta-Analysis. Neural Plast. 2020 Nov 25;2020:8842110. doi: 10.1155/2020/8842110. PMID: 33299396; PMCID: PMC7710408.

Makrantonaki E, Zouboulis CC: Androgens and ageing of the skin. Curr Opin Endocrinol Diabetes Obes 2009;16:240-245.

Marsh ML, Oliveira MN, Vieira-Potter VJ. Adipocyte Metabolism and Health after the Menopause: The Role of Exercise. Nutrients. 2023 Jan 14;15(2):444. doi: 10.3390/nu15020444. PMID: 36678314; PMCID: PMC9862030.

Mattson MP, Moehl K, Ghena N, Schmaedick M, Cheng A. Melby, M. 2005. Vasomotor symptom prevalence and language of menopause in Japan. Menopause, 12 (3), 250–257. URL (abstract): https://www.ncbi.nlm.nih.gov/pubmed/15879913

Melby, M. 2007. Chilliness: A vasomotor symptom in Japan. Menopause, 14 (4), 752–759. URL (abstract): https://www.ncbi.nlm.nih.gov/sites/pubmed/17538512 (accessed 09.10.2007).

Memar P, Faradji F. A Novel Multi-Class EEG-Based Sleep Stage Classification System. IEEE Trans Neural Syst Rehabil Eng. 2018 Jan;26(1):84-95.

Mishra N, Mishra VN, Devanshi. Exercise beyond menopause: Dos and Don'ts. J Midlife Health. 2011 Jul;2(2):51-6. doi:

10.4103/0976-7800.92524. PMID: 22408332; PMCID: PMC3296386.

Mohamad Ishak NN, Jamani NA, Mohd Arifin SR, Abdul Hadi A, Abd Aziz KH. Exploring women's perceptions and experiences of menopause among East Coast Malaysian women. Malays Fam Physician. 2021 Feb 1;16(1):84-92. doi: 10.51866/oa1098. PMID: 33948146; PMCID: PMC8088743.

Mosconi L, Berti V, Dyke J, Schelbaum E, Jett S, Loughlin L, Jang G, Rahman A, Hristov H, Pahlajani S, Andrews R, Matthews D, Etingin O, Ganzer C, de Leon M, Isaacson R, Brinton RD. Menopause impacts human brain structure, connectivity, energy metabolism, and amyloid-beta deposition. Sci Rep. 2021 Jun 9;11(1):10867. doi: 10.1038/s41598-021-90084-y. PMID: 34108509; PMCID: PMC8190071.

Nappi RE, Palacios S. Impact of vulvovaginal atrophy on sexual health and quality of life at postmenopause. Climacteric. 2014;17:3–9. [PubMed] [Google Scholar].

Nat Rev Neurosci. 2020 Aug;21(8):445. doi: 10.1038/s41583-020-0342-y.

Nelson H Haney E Humphrey L et al. Management of menopause-related symptoms. Evidence Report/Technology Assessment 120.Agency for Healthcare Research and Quality, Rockville, MD 2005.

Nelson, L. R., & Bulun, S. E. (2001). Oestrogen production and action. Journal of the American Academy of Dermatology, 45(3), S116-S124.

Newson L, Rymer J. The dangers of compounded bioidentical hormone replacement therapy. Br J Gen Pract. 2019 Oct

31;69(688):540-541. doi: 10.3399/bjgp19X706169. PMID: 31672802; PMCID: PMC6808563.

Papatriantafyllou E, Efthymiou D, Zoumbaneas E, Popescu CA, Vassilopoulou E. Sleep Deprivation: Effects on Weight Loss and Weight Loss Maintenance. Nutrients. 2022 Apr 8;14(8):1549. doi: 10.3390/nu14081549. PMID: 35458110; PMCID: PMC9031614.

Pourhadi N, MÃ¸rch L S, Holm E A, Torp-Pedersen C, Meaidi A. Menopausal hormone therapy and dementia: nationwide, nested case-control study BMJ 2023; 381 :e072770 doi:10.1136/bmj-2022-072770

Quatresooz P, Pierard GE: Downgrading skin climacteric aging by hormone replacement therapy. Expert Rev Dermatol 2007;2:373-376.

Rajapakse, C.S., et al. Effect of Low-Intensity Vibration on Bone Strength, Microstructure, and Adiposity in Pre-Osteoporotic Postmenopausal Women: A Randomized Placebo-Controlled Trial. (2021).

Rees, M., et al. (2020). Management of the Menopause. Postgraduate Medical Journal, 96(1132), 40–47. doi: 10.1136/postgradmedj-2019-136659.

Richards, J. S. (1980). Maturation of ovarian follicles: actions and interactions of pituitary and ovarian hormones on follicular cell differentiation. Physiological reviews, 60(1), 51-89.

Romani WA, Gallicchio L, Flaws JA. The association between physical activity and hot flash severity, frequency, and duration in mid-life women. Am J Hum Biol. 2009 Jan-Feb;21(1):127-9. doi: 10.1002/ajhb.20834. PMID: 18942715; PMCID: PMC2753173

Salehi B, Machin L, Monzote L, Sharifi-Rad J, Ezzat SM, Salem MA, Merghany RM, El Mahdy NM, K?I?ç CS, Sytar O, Sharifi-Rad M, Sharopov F, Martins N, Martorell M, Cho WC. Therapeutic Potential of Quercetin: New Insights and Perspectives for Human Health. ACS Omega. 2020 May 14;5(20):11849-11872. doi: 10.1021/acsomega.0c01818. PMID: 32478277; PMCID: PMC7254783.

Salpeter, S.R., Walsh, J.M., Ormiston, T.M. et al. (2006). Meta-analysis: effect of hormone replacement therapy on components of the metabolic syndrome in postmenopausal women. Diabetes, Obesity and Metabolism, 8, pp. 538-554.

Santana-Gálvez J, Cisneros-Zevallos L, Jacobo-Velázquez DA. Chlorogenic Acid: Recent Advances on Its Dual Role as a Food Additive and a Nutraceutical against Metabolic Syndrome. Molecules. 2017 Feb 26;22(3):358. doi: 10.3390/molecules22030358. PMID: 28245635; PMCID: PMC6155416.

Santoro, N., & Randolph, J. F. (2011). Reproductive hormones and the menopause transition. Obstetrics and Gynecology Clinics, 38(3), 455-466.

Santoro, N., et al. (2016). Menopausal Hormone Therapy and Women's Health. Endocrine Reviews, 37(6), 584–607. doi: 10.1210/er.2016-1067.

Shumaker SA, Legault C, Rapp SR, Thal L, Wallace RB, Ockene JK, Hendrix SL, Jones BN 3rd, Assaf AR, Jackson RD, Kotchen JM, Wassertheil-Smoller S, Wactawski-Wende J; WHIMS Investigators. Estrogen plus progestin and the incidence of dementia and mild cognitive impairment in postmenopausal women: the Women's Health Initiative Memory Study: a randomized controlled trial. JAMA. 2003 May 28;289(20):2651-62. doi: 10.1001/jama.289.20.2651. PMID: 12771112.

Simpkins JW, Brown K, Bae S, Ratka A. Role of ethnicity in the expression of features of hot flashes. Maturitas. 2009 Aug 20;63(4):341-6. doi: 10.1016/j.maturitas.2009.06.002. Epub 2009 Jul 9. PMID: 19592184; PMCID: PMC7050441.

Singh A, Kaur S, Walia I. A historical perspective on menopause and menopausal age. Bull Indian Inst Hist Med Hyderabad. 2002 Jul-Dec;32(2):121-35. PMID: 15981376.

Singh, V., Sivakami, M. (2020). Normality, Freedom, and Distress: Listening to the Menopausal Experiences of Indian Women of Haryana. In: Bobel, C., Winkler, I.T., Fahs, B., Hasson, K.A., Kissling, E.A., Roberts, TA. (eds) The Palgrave Handbook of Critical Menstruation Studies. Palgrave Macmillan, Singapore. https://doi.org/10.1007/978-981-15-0614-7_70.

Smith RL, Flaws JA, Gallicchio L. Does quitting smoking decrease the risk of midlife hot flashes? A longitudinal analysis. Maturitas. 2015 Sep;82(1):123-7. doi: 10.1016/j.maturitas.2015.06.029. Epub 2015 Jun 22. PMID: 26149340; PMCID: PMC4546860.

Soules, M. R., Sherman, S., Parrott, E., Rebar, R., Santoro, N., Utian, W., ... & Rebar, R. (2001). Executive summary: Stages of reproductive ageing workshop (STRAW). Fertility and sterility, 76(5), 874-878.

Sözen T, Öz???k L, Ba?aran NÇ. An overview and management of osteoporosis. Eur J Rheumatol. 2017 Mar;4(1):46-56. doi: 10.5152/eurjrheum.2016.048. Epub 2016 Dec 30. PMID: 28293453; PMCID: PMC5335887.

Speroff, L., Fritz, M. A., & Cibula, D. (2018). Clinical Gynaecologic Endocrinology and Infertility. Wolters Kluwer.

Sternfeld B, Dugan S. Physical activity and health during the menopausal transition. Obstet Gynecol Clin North Am. 2011 Sep;38(3):537-66. doi: 10.1016/j.ogc.2011.05.008. PMID: 21961719; PMCID: PMC3270074.

Syan R, Brucker BM. Guideline of guidelines: urinary incontinence. BJU Int. 2016 Jan;117(1):20-33. doi: 10.1111/bju.13187. Epub 2015 Jul 1. PMID: 26033093.

The Centre for Men's Health. "What Are Normal Male Testosterone Levels?" Centre for Men's Health, 4 Oct. 2023, www.centreformenshealth.co.uk/what-are-normal-male-testosterone-levels#:~:text=International%20medical%20opinions%20vary&text=The%20British%20Society%20for%20Sexual,testosterone%20below%200.225%20nmol%2Fl.

The Perception of the Menopause and the Climacteric among Women in Hong Kong and Southern China, Preventive Medicine, Volume 24, Issue 3, 1995, Pages 245-248, ISSN 0091-7435,

Thornton MJ. Estrogens and aging skin. Dermatoendocrinol. 2013 Apr 1;5(2):264-70. doi: 10.4161/derm.23872. PMID: 24194966; PMCID: PMC3772914.

Thurston RC, Ewing LJ, Low CA, Christie AJ, Levine MD. Behavioral weight loss for the management of menopausal hot flashes: a pilot study. Menopause. 2015 Jan;22(1):59-65. doi: 10.1097/GME.0000000000000274. PMID: 24977456; PMCID: PMC4270932.

Tortora, G. J., & Derrickson, B. (2017). Principles of Anatomy and Physiology (15th ed.). Wiley.

Tu KN, Lie JD, Wan CKV, Cameron M, Austel AG, Nguyen JK, Van K, Hyun D. Osteoporosis: A Review of Treatment Options. P T. 2018 Feb;43(2):92-104. PMID: 29386866; PMCID: PMC5768298.

UK, NHS. NHS Choices, NHS, 30 Dec. 2021, www.nhs.uk/conditions/vaginal-dryness/.

Vander, A. J., Sherman, J. H., & Luciano, D. S. (2001). Human Physiology: The Mechanisms of Body Function (8th ed.). McGraw-Hill.

Vogel, S., Schwabe, L. Learning and memory under stress: implications for the classroom. npj Science Learn 1, 16011 (2016). https://doi.org/10.1038/npjscilearn.2016.11

Welton S, Minty R, O'Driscoll T, Willms H, Poirier D, Madden S, Kelly L. Intermittent fasting and weight loss: Systematic review. Can Fam Physician. 2020 Feb;66(2):117-125. PMID: 32060194; PMCID: PMC7021351.

WHO. "Menopause." World Health Organization, World Health Organization, 2022, www.who.int/news-room/fact-sheets/detail/menopause.

Zilberstein, Inga. "5 Benefits of Bioidentical Hormone Replacement Therapy." 5 Benefits of Bioidentical Hormone Replacement Therapy: Inga Zilberstein, MD: Gynecology, 2023, www.drzilberstein.com/blog/5-benefits-of-bioidentical-hormone-replacement-therapy.

Zurlo F, Larson K, Bogardus C, Ravussin E. Skeletal muscle metabolism is a major determinant of resting energy expenditure. J Clin Invest. 1990 Nov;86(5):1423-7. doi: 10.1172/JCI114857. PMID: 2243122; PMCID: PMC296885.

INDEX

C

D

E

F

S

sarcopenia 99, 116, 132
serotonin 61, 62, 64, 65, 91, 234
skin 17, 19, 29, 39, 51, 53-62, 98, 107, 122, 123, 249, 274, 275, 278, 280, 283
sleep diary 202-204
sleep disruption 198
smoking 56, 58, 84, 89, 182, 184, 195, 233, 253, 282
soy 110-112
spiritual 15, 16
sugar 27, 29, 94, 95, 103, 104, 112, 115, 132, 212, 217, 233
sun 56-58
surgery 24, 70, 73, 85, 122
synovial 88

T

testosterone 29, 30, 37, 38, 40, 43, 77, 81, 92, 99, 130-133, 249, 271, 272, 278, 283
thought distortions 164, 187, 189, 192
turmeric 113
typical menopausal symptoms 13, 38, 39

U

urinary symptom diary 258
uterus 25, 26, 33, 34, 47, 48, 70, 71

V

vaginismus 251
vitamin D(3) 15, 77, 81, 83, 113, 115, 212, 218, 233

Printed in Dunstable, United Kingdom